FORAGING
FOR BEGINNERS

MONA GREENY

Table of Contents

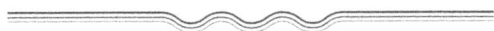

FORAGING FOR BEGINNERS
Identifying Mushrooms in North America

FORAGING FOR BEGINNERS
Identifying Medicinal Plants in North America

FORAGING FOR BEGINNERS
Identifying Fruits, Nuts and Seeds in North America

FORAGING
FOR BEGINNERS

Identifying Mushrooms in North America

MONA GREENY

Introduction

Foraging, or gathering of food, was one of the primary means our hunter-gatherer ancestors met their food requirements. They hunted animals and gathered plants and plant parts, including roots, berries, and fruits from nature, to sustain their food requirements. It seems like our ancestors valued the importance of eating naturally grown food far more than we do today. Of course, there is no denying the fact that our ancestors had no choice but to dip into the lap of nature for their food needs.

And yet, it is time for our 'ultra-civilized' humanity to learn something from our hunter-gatherer ancestors and reach out to nature and take what we need from her. The trick is to remember to take from Mother Nature what we need and not to fulfill our greed. Foraging for food is an excellent start to reconnect with nature and learn to value what she offers to us.

The History of Foraging

In the prehistoric times, our ancestors would pick wild, edible plants for their food. Depending on the season and type of food foraged, they were consumed immediately or preserved for later use, especially for the times when food would be scarce.

For example, some roots and nuts were collected and preserved for future use, while fresh fruit and vegetables were eaten immediately. Our nomadic ancestors extensively used foraging. During the Neolithic Age, our nomadic ancestors had learned to cultivate the land and domesticate animals.

Consequently, they were able to 'settle down' in one place instead of having to move from place to place in search of food and shelter. Agriculture slowly but surely became a prominent way of food production for human beings. As we embraced civilization and with the tremendous growth and development of agriculture, food gathering turned into a structured format called harvesting.

Over time, harvesting turned into economic activity, and the concept of harvesting was made into a structured and regulated process. Despite the expansion of agriculture, wild foraging continued to help the underprivileged and the poor sections of society to supplement their often insufficient diet.

Also, this way of finding food continued to be popular among people who had not yet developed systematic societies. Slowly, as time passed, and standards of living increased across all sections of society, foraging in the wild became seen as an activity of leisure, especially in the West. Most city-dwellers would visit the countryside just to spend time foraging and harnessing its multiple benefits.

Foraging was also used extensively by us during times of food scarcity. For example, during World War II, poverty and hunger were rife in most parts of the globe. Foraging is what helped many people survive those difficult times. Also, during that time, important supplements such as Vitamin C were not easily available as trade restrictions were imposed. Coffee was another item that had trade restrictions. The daily dose of Vitamin C was obtained by eating rose hips that were foraged, and dandelion and acorn roots were popular replacements for coffee.

In the 20th century, foraging was an important element of the 'hippie movement' symbolizing the return of human beings to nature. Also, the activity was seen as a form of social engagement and helped to develop awareness of a conscious attitude towards the consumption of food.

Of late, the activity of foraging for wild plants has gained immense popularity as people invest in it both for fun as well as to harness the power of eating local and organically grown fresh ingredients. So, what does the activity of foraging entail?

Foraging involves searching for, identifying, and collecting food and natural ingredients from the wild, including nuts, roots, herbs, berries, plants, mushrooms, and sometimes, shellfish too. Foraging brings you closer to nature as you try to understand the natural environment and learn to respect what nature gives you even as you get the opportunity to eat healthy and nutritious food.

Benefits of Foraging

Benefits of foraging are numerous and investing time and energy on this activity will help you harness many of these advantages, which include:

Foraging gets you closer to nature - As an urban-dweller, surrounded by tall skyscrapers offer great convenience for modern-day living. But, urban-dwelling have its flip side to it, including the pain of choking traffic, insufficient amounts of fresh air, living in claustrophobic accommodations, and more.

To get out of this kind of life occasionally can be a great way to rejuvenate and refresh yourself by harnessing the power of nature. Foraging helps you do just that. In fact, in the US, you might not have to go very far from your place of stay to indulge in some amount of foraging. You could find edible plants and mushrooms closer than you think.

Moreover, getting outdoors means you are investing in your health through another way, namely great outdoor exercise. Hiking and walking the trails of the wild is a great way to get your quota of exercise even as you gather free, nutritious food ingredients.

Another benefit of being outdoors is that being out in the sunlight gives your body the time needed to build up its Vitamin D reservoir naturally. You might get the opportunity to get rid of one artificial supplement from your medicine cabinet.

Access to free, organic, healthy, tasty, and nutritious food - Food ingredients picked from the wild offer far more nutrition and health than those picked off from store shelves. For example, the leafy greens of the wild dandelion offer multiple times more phytonutrients than the leafy greens from store-bought spinach or kale. Also, edible crab apples picked from the wild are known to be more nutritious than the common apples purchased from any supermarket.

You also understand that foraging costs you no money. The food you gather is yours for free. The only thing you will spend is your time and energy in return for which you will get amply compensated with good health and happiness. Of course, your time is valuable, which is why it makes sense to forage for expensive ingredients like chanterelle mushrooms, pine nuts, etc.

Not only do you get expensive ingredients for free, but you also get to try new flavors. All of us know how store-bought food tastes, either sweet, savory, bland, or a mixture of these flavors. Our taste buds are exposed to the same kind of taste day in and day out and have lost their ability to associate themselves with new flavors.

For example, bitterness is a taste that our tongue has gotten unaccustomed to. We have learned to disassociate bitter taste with pleasantness. However, bitter herbs have been one of the most common ways of detoxing our bodies since prehistoric times. For example, dandelion is a bitter plant offering outstanding health benefits. Eating foraged dandelions is a wonderful way to get our taste buds to reconnect bitterness with pleasantness.

Also, some ingredients like some wild mushrooms cannot be bought in stores. Foraging in the wild is the only way you can taste the flavors of certain wild mushrooms. Therefore, foraging gives you an opportunity to taste new, unique, and untried flavors.

Contributing to nature's sustainability - This wonderful activity helps you connect with nature. The modern world is increasingly moving away from nature driven by technological advances and excessive human intervention in nature's cycles for the sake of convenience and luxury. After all, it is so much easier to pick up harvested and cleaned ingredients off the store shelves. However, we don't get the opportunity to see how these ingredients are grown, harvested, and transported to your local store. We only see the end-result that is convenient for us.

Foraging in the wild not only provides you with organically-grown and chemical-free ingredients but also those that have used only rainwater or other forms of naturally-available water to grow. Harvesting these wild ingredients does not use fossil fuels of any kind, which means the carbon footprint is almost nil when you go out foraging in the wild. Therefore, you participate directly and actively in maintaining sustainability in nature.

Foraging helps you reconnect with nature. You can watch and indulge in the joy of seeing wild dandelions and mushrooms flourishing in their natural environment. As you watch the various fruit and flowers blossom in front of your eyes, the beauty of nature is revealed to you, and you will feel a close connection with nature.

Foraging improves your overall well-being by helping you connect with nature so that you can see not only the beauty she has to offer, but how easy it is to lead a simple but content life. There is almost a spiritual awakening that you are likely to feel when you delve deep into the activity of mushroom foraging.

You can see how many benefits foraging offers you. And yet, there are some important points to keep in mind when you are foraging. Some hazards have to be taken care of to prevent untoward incidents. So, what are the hazards of foraging?

Hazards of Foraging

The risks of foraging include:

Eating a poisonous or harmful plant. The biggest challenge in foraging is learning to know the differences between nutritious plants and poisonous ones because both can look similar. It takes a discerning eye to know the difference and to make sure you don't end up eating something you shouldn't. Not all harmful plants have fatal effects.

Some of them could make you sick. In fact, some of the plants foraged could make you sick not because of their inherent chemical or biological properties but because they have been contaminated by animal waste or chemical residues in the soil or any other thing.

Note of caution: Many mushrooms look very similar and can be difficult to tell apart. Some can be deadly. If you are unsure, don't eat them!

Causing harm to the environment. Inexperienced and insensitive foragers can cause a lot of harm to the environment, knowingly or unknowingly. Foraging has to be done ethically so that all the species can grow again and survive. It takes time and effort to learn to forage ethically, ensuring you are not stripping an entire area of its edible foliage.

In such conditions, invasive species of plants quickly take over the area, making it impossible for the edible species to survive. Unethical foraging can result in damaging the delicate balance of nature in that area. Also, inexperienced foragers can trample the ground, crush the plants and crucial germs and microbes, damage the topsoil, and disrupt the environment in irreversible ways.

Dealing with unfamiliar ingredients. Another interesting aspect of foraged plants and plant parts is that many edible and safe plants could be tough, bitter, or indigestible unless cooked correctly. Therefore, if you go on foraging expeditions with a lack of knowledge, you could end up with a lot of edible things in your hand, which will ultimately be wasted.

Foraging illegally. Not all the wild spaces are available for foraging. Some of the state and federal parks in the US do not allow foraging. So, if you are caught foraging in such places, it is illegal, and you could be booked for it. Even in places where foraging is legal, there are limits to what part and how much of an edible plant you can take.

In many places, there are no clear demarcations separating lands on which foraging is legal and where it is illegal. So, it is possible that you unwittingly move into an area where foraging is illegal and such situations could put you in unpleasant situations.

Therefore, you must learn everything you need to know about foraging for a particular species, as well as knowing what is legal and what is not. Only when you are certain of your knowledge and know your lessons well, can you enjoy the magical activity of foraging even as you harness its multiple benefits.

So, go on, and begin your ride starting right at the basics of understanding mushrooms and diving deep into detailed explanations of certain wild mushrooms that are found in abundance in North America.

Chapter One

Understanding Mushrooms

A common misconception among people is that mushrooms are vegetables. No, they are not. They belong to the Fungi Kingdom. Why are they not vegetables? Because mushrooms do not come from edible plants. One of the primary characteristic features of plants is that they contain an element called chlorophyll, which helps them convert sunlight into carbohydrates through the process of photosynthesis. Mushrooms do not have chlorophyll, and therefore, cannot photosynthesize. Mushrooms steal carbohydrates from other plants.

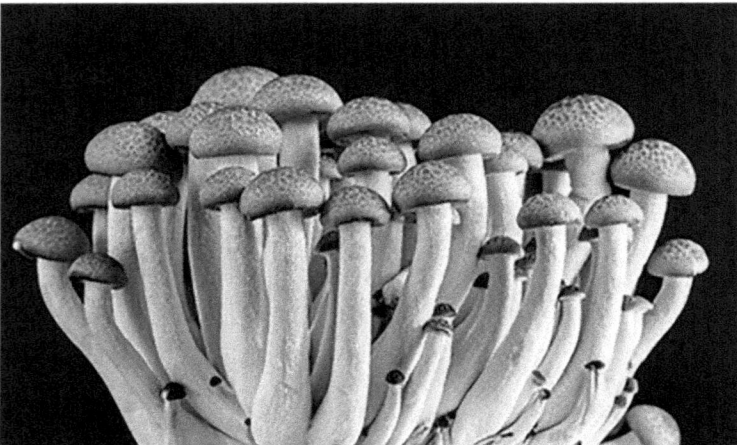

As mushrooms belong to the fungi kingdom, it makes sense to learn a bit about fungi in general before we focus on mushrooms specifically. Fungi are divided into three separate categories depending on the relationship with their parent plant. All three categories of mushrooms exist.

Mushrooms start life in the form of a white fluff referred to as 'mycelium' from under the ground. The mycelium is a collection of fungal threads that sprout into potential mushrooms when the conditions are conducive. Mushrooms are actually the fruiting bodies of a much larger fungus that grows underground.

In the wild, mycelium can remain safe and secure for a very long time under the ground. When circumstances are favorable for its growth, then the mycelium sprouts and grows into mushrooms. Favorable circumstances include the right humidity and temperature, as well as the availability of food.

Under such circumstances, the mycelium form buds which seek out sunlight. These buds represent the birth of mushrooms. The buds, which are usually small white balls, grow rapidly into a proper mushroom. The cap then opens up, and millions of spores (minuscule seeds) are dropped into the atmosphere. The wind spreads these spores, and when they land on the ground, these minuscule seeds start forming another mycelium.

Understanding the Parts of a Mushroom

There are essentially two parts in mushrooms, namely the mycelium, which grows under the ground, and the umbrella-shaped part called the fruit or sporophore, which grows above the ground. The fruit begins as a small button, which then grows into a stalk at a rapid pace because it absorbs plenty of water very fast.

The cap at the end of the stalk slowly unfolds like an umbrella. Under this cap, small plates called gills can be seen. The cap also has small spores or seeds on them. These seeds are blown away by the wind, and when they land on the ground elsewhere, they grow into new mycelium. Medicinal mushrooms are sometimes referred to as toadstools. Let us look at some of the important parts of the mushrooms in a bit of detail:

- The cap - Located at the top of the mushroom and shaped like an umbrella, the cap is the most obvious part of the mushroom. Mushroom caps come in different colors, although the most common colors include white, brown, or yellow.

- Gills - Also referred to as teeth or pores, gills that look similar to fish gills, are found under the cap.

- Ring - Also known as the annulus, the ring is the remaining part of the mushroom veil after the gills have been pushed through the cap.

- Stem - Also called stipe, the stem of a mushroom is the tall stalk that holds the cap above the ground.

- Volva - The volva is the protective veil that remains connected to the ground and the mushroom after the fruiting body has sprouted out from the ground. As the mushroom grows from the mycelium, it breaks through the volva.

Types of Mushrooms

There are more than 10,00o known species of mushrooms all around the globe. Although this number might seem huge, experts in the field of mycology believe that there are many thousands more undiscovered by human beings. All these known species of mushrooms are typically categorized into four types, namely saprophytes or saprotrophs, mycorrhizae, parasites, and endophytes. Let us look at each type in a bit of detail.

Saprophytes

Saprophytic mushrooms live and thrive on dead organic matter such as dead wood, fallen leaves, and roots of plants and trees. Saprophytes extract minerals and carbon dioxide from the hosts to survive and grow. You would find many medicinal and gourmet mushrooms in this category, including:

- White button mushrooms - One of the most common mushrooms found in all the supermarkets around the world. It is a highly popular mushroom in the US with statistics showing that an average American consumes about 3 pounds of white button mushrooms annually.

- Oyster mushrooms - known for its cholesterol-reducing benefits.

- Shiitake mushrooms - highly popular for its taste as well as medicinal value.

- Turkey tail - The only way this saprophytic mushroom is consumable is as a tea as it is too tough to be edible and digestible. And yet, it is one of the most well-studied mushroom species.

- A few species of morels - For example, Morchella angusticeps and Morchella esculenta are highly delicious, but elusive mushrooms are a forager's delight.

- Reishi (a mushroom valued highly in Chinese medicine)

Saprophytic mushrooms are also referred to as decomposers. These kinds of mushrooms release enzymes and acids onto decaying matter breaking down dead tissues into small molecules that can be easily absorbed. Therefore, dead and decaying plants, wood, and animals become food for saprophytes.

Imagine the world without saprophytes. It would be filled with dead and decaying matter left unprocessed to putrefy. Saprophytic mushrooms are natural cleaners of our earth ridding it of dead and decaying matter even as they turn into some of the most delicious mushrooms filled with medicinal benefits too.

Parasites

Parasites live on and extract nutrients from living plants and trees, which is the reason they are referred to as murderer mushrooms. With one-sided force, parasitic mushrooms infect the host and finally destroy it completely. When the trees and plants on which parasites live die, the saprophytic mushrooms use these dead resources for their growth and development. Some examples of parasitic mushrooms are:

- Honey mushrooms - are the fruiting bodies of honey fungus have a fruity and nutty flavor and are loved by many mushroom fans.

- Caterpillar fungus - This fungus preys on insects and is considered to be one of the most valuable parasites on our planet. Although in strictly technical terms, the fruiting body of this parasitic fungus is considered an ascocarp, a phylum (a subset(of the Fungi Kingdom, most people refer to them as a mushroom, and one of the most expensive ones. Caterpillar fungus is restricted to the Himalayan regions.

- Lion's Mane - This type of mushroom has spiny teeth instead of the traditional mushroom cap.

Mycorrhiza

Mycorrhizal mushrooms have a symbiotic relationship with their living hosts. They grow on the roots of living trees. They take nutrients and carbohydrates from the host and pass on minerals, moisture, and other essential elements in return, which helps in the growth and development of the root system of the trees. Mycorrhizal mushrooms tend to grow faster and bigger than the other types of mushrooms. Also, mycorrhizal mushrooms are not easy to cultivate and are only found in the wild. Here are some popular examples of mycorrhizal mushrooms:

- Porcini mushrooms - are commonly used in sauces and soups. They can grow to very large sizes.

- Matsutake mushrooms - offers great aroma and flavor in cooking.

- Truffle mushrooms - These gourmet ingredients are an expensive luxury item.

- Chanterelles - found in many continents including North America, chanterelles are prized edible mushrooms.

Endophytes

Endophytic mushrooms are categorized separately because of their unique features. Like parasites, endophytes invade the body of their host. But, there is no harm caused to the host body. Instead, the host body gets the benefits as in the case of mycorrhizal mushrooms even though it is not clear how the beneficial partnership is formed.

Also, unlike mycorrhizal mushrooms, endophytic mushrooms can be cultivated. The uniqueness of this class of mushrooms lies in the mysterious nature of the symbiotic relationship between the host and the fungi.

Life Cycle of Mushrooms

Mushrooms have a distinctive life cycle that is dependent on the environment in which they grow and the size to which they grow.

The small-sized mushrooms take about one day to grow, whereas the larger ones can take up to 3-4 days to fully mature. A steady flow of moisture and dampness is essential for the healthy growth of mushrooms and for them to complete their life cycle successfully.

You already know that mushrooms are not vegetables but are the fruits of fungi that grow everywhere. Mushrooms can grow on the ground, on dead tree stumps, and on living trees and plants. Mushrooms release spores from gills, teeth, or pores found on the underside of their caps. Spores are similar to seeds that have the potential to grow into more mushrooms. Every mushroom can produce numerous spores that get separated from the parent mushrooms and spread themselves all over the forest.

Each spore is a single cell that can be male or female. Many male spores and many female spores join together to form male and female hyphae. When the male and female hyphae join together, they begin the process of producing mycelium.

Mycelium is the stage in the life cycle of a mushroom wherein it takes a visible form for the first time. You can imagine mycelium to be the equivalent of the roots of a plant or tree. Mycelium is a web-like network formed under the ground that is rooted. However, mycelium can also branch out like the branches of a tree. Mycelium is what provides food and nutrients to the fungi to start producing the fruiting bodies or the mushrooms.

The next stage in the life cycle of a mushroom is the formation of hyphal knots. It is the first point on the surface of the mycelium at which the pinhead or baby mushrooms start to sprout. Hyphal knots are just points, and when pinheads form on the hyphal knots is when you can see the baby mushrooms begin to take visible shape. Not all the pinheads that are formed on hyphal knots grow into mushrooms. Some of them stop growing. In fact, many of the pinheads in a mycelium colony stop growing.

Benefits and Uses of Mushrooms

Mushrooms are a truly amazing variety of food. They are great substitutes for meat, which is one of the primary reasons for the increasing popularity of this fungus among the nouveau vegans of the West. In addition, these low-calories ingredients (most varieties of mushrooms are low in calories) offer a multitude of health benefits that are hard to counter. Let us look at some of the benefits of mushrooms in a bit of detail.

Mushrooms are rich in antioxidants to keep you young. Mushrooms have a high concentration of two important antioxidants, namely glutathione and ergothioneine. Studies have shown that when both these antioxidants work in tandem, their ability to keep physiological stress affecting the aging process at bay is increased manifold.

Physiological effects of aging, such as the formation of wrinkles, reduction in bone density, etc. are minimized by the combined effects of glutathione and ergothioneine, both of which are found in abundance in mushrooms. The abundance of antioxidants also helps in boosting your immune system by protecting your body against the harmful effects of free radicals.

Mushrooms also protect your brain and brain cells. The same two antioxidants, including glutathione and ergothioneine, are also believed to be effective in preventing Alzheimer's and Parkinson's, according to some studies conducted by Pennsylvania University. The researchers who conducted these studies claim that eating mushrooms five times a week reduces the risk of neurological illnesses related to the brain and nervous system. Additionally, mushrooms can help to build your memory skills too.

Mushrooms are good for the health of your heart. The glutamate ribonucleotides present in mushrooms are an excellent salt substitute. The savory taste of this naturally-occurring chemical compound in mushrooms ensures you get the taste of salt without affecting your blood pressure and associated risk of heart diseases. The meaty taste of mushrooms makes them a great supplement for meats minus the side-effects on cholesterol and fat.

Mushrooms contain plenty of lean proteins which help in burning excess fat and cholesterol in your body. These fungi have negligible amounts of cholesterol and fat. The beta-glucan and chitin found in mushrooms are excellent sources of fiber, which help to keep your cholesterol levels in check. Therefore, mushrooms apply a multi-pronged approach to keeping your fat and cholesterol levels healthy.

Mushrooms build bone strength. Calcium-rich mushrooms are excellent to strengthen your bones, thereby reducing the risks of bone-related disorders such as joint pain, osteoporosis, etc.

Therefore, mushrooms with their spongy and meat-like texture are an excellent addition to your daily diet. There was a time in history when mushrooms were considered exotic ingredients. In fact, the ancient Egyptians preserved these fungi for royalty only while the ancient Romans preserved them for their soldiers as they believed mushrooms helped improve the physical strength and stamina of their warriors. Today, they are easily available off the market shelves.

Foraging for Mushrooms in the US

Foraging for mushrooms in the United States is gaining popularity for the following reasons:

- The amazing health benefits offered by this wonder ingredient.

- The advantages of participating in foraging.

- The availability of several thousand varieties of mushrooms in the country.

Most of these several thousand varieties are 'edible' though many of them are too fibrous and cannot really be digested. About a few hundred from this big collection are poisonous. That still leaves you a large number of mushroom varieties to choose from for your foraging activities.

Despite the favorable numbers in respect of edible, non-poisonous varieties of mushrooms, you must learn all the important aspects of mushroom foraging to ensure healthy and ethical pickings. Using guesswork to choose the right kind of mushrooms to forage for is a complete no-no. There have been multiple cases of mushroom poisoning, some of which resulted in fatality too.

One of the most significant dangers in mushroom foraging is the similarity between edible and poisonous varieties. A common example is the poisonous "green-spored parasol" variety of mushrooms that appear in the US after rainfalls during the summer and fall seasons. When this mushroom is at the developing stage, it looks a lot like the white-button mushroom variety found in abundance in grocery stores.

Two more commonly mistaken couples include:

- The tasty and popular morel mushrooms have toxic lookalikes in Gyromitra, Helvella, and Verpa species.

- Poisonous jack-o'-lantern mushrooms look very similar to the exotic chanterelle mushrooms.

The most common reason for making mistakes while discerning between edible and poisonous varieties of mushrooms is the lack of sufficient knowledge, especially by novice foragers. Many inexperienced and overly eager foragers tend to take an 'I-know-enough' attitude with regard to learning this crucial aspect of mushroom foraging. They forget that looks can be easily deceiving and end up committing rookie errors needlessly endangering their health.

Here are some important tips to follow to prevent unnecessary mishaps while foraging for mushrooms:

• Be part of a support group collectively referred to as mycology or fungi group. Many such self-help groups are mushrooming all over the US, and taking the advice and recommendations of the reputed and qualified experts heading any of these groups can add value to your learning and experience in mushroom foraging.

- Get yourself a local guide and map that shows wild mushrooms growing in the specific area that you are foraging in.

- Learn to identify the genus of the mushroom you found by looking at vital identification elements such as the spore print, the stem, the surface on which the mushroom grows, and the stem base. (these elements are covered in separate chapters in this book).

- Always carry two containers to collect foraged mushrooms. Put the positively identified mushrooms in one container and the ones you are uncertain about in the second one.

You need to take extra caution if you are taking your pet, especially a dog, with you on your foraging trip. Pets lead the list in terms of succumbing to the effects of poisonous mushrooms.

Mushroom foraging and picking involve a wide range of emotions and experiences right from the focus and concentration needed to look for the right ones to the care taken to pick them the right way to the delight and joy of eating them. Mushroom foraging is one of the best forms of mindfulness and can be a soothing balm to a troubled mind.

Other than the above slightly off-beat philosophical approach to mushroom foraging, it is also one of the most fun and highly productive activities to engage in. So, go on, read on, and find more tips and a lot of help on how you can begin the journey of foraging for mushrooms. This book includes a few simple recipes for some of the wild mushrooms.

Chapter Two

Things to Do and Obtain Before the Start of Mushroom Foraging

There are very few items and equipment needed to start off your journey of mushroom foraging. However, some elements and resources are critical to have before you start out. This chapter is dedicated to giving you an overview of what you need to do and have before you begin your love affair with mushrooms in North America.

Get Educated

One of the biggest fears and mistakes that novice mushroom hunters make is to end up consuming a wrong species of mushroom, resulting in disastrous, and sometimes even fatal, outcomes. This fear and anxiety are well-founded, and the only way you can overcome this obstacle is by educating yourself on mushrooms, its effects, benefits, and the bad effects of the bad ones.

A common warning-laced adage among mushroom foragers goes something like this, "There are bold mushroom foragers, and there are 'old' mushroom hunters. However, you can never find a bold as well as an old mushroom forager."

Mushroom-related fatalities are quite rare in North America, thankfully. According to the National Poison Data System, there are not more than three mushroom-related deaths each year in the United States. However, there are many more people who experience nasty side-effects of consuming the wrong kinds of mushrooms. These side-effects range from mild nausea and vomiting to liver and malfunctioning, requiring lifetime medical support of some sort.

Mixing up edible, safe mushrooms with poisonous ones are the commonest mistakes made by novice mushroom hunters. Therefore, it is imperative that before you go foraging for mushrooms, you familiarize yourself thoroughly with regard to the characteristic features of the mushrooms you are hunting for. A good-quality mushroom-identifying book is the best way to achieve this goal.

A must-have is a guidebook that features the mushrooms of the specific geographical area you want to go foraging in. The localized guidebook is essential because the distribution of mushrooms varies from place to place.

A single-page key is detailing the parts of the mushrooms in your specific area. This one-page guide will give you a ballpark idea of whether you are looking at an expected variety of fungus, or it is a completely unfamiliar one.

Other than the above two essential things to carry on your mushroom-foraging journey, some things that might be a great but not necessary thing to have on you include:

- A general primer on mushroom foraging in North America, not specific to your region. These kinds of general books are great and useful additions to your library, especially if you are the kind who loves to forage even while traveling.

- A mushroom-identifying app is also a great way to ensure you don't end up collecting the wrong kinds of fungus. Although this kind of app is not essential, it might be a good idea to have one installed on your phone so that you can accurately identify any unfamiliar mushrooms.

Getting educated on mushroom foraging does not mean you have to learn by rote all the things you need to know. It only means you can more or less identify the wrong ones and have the good sense not to be unduly overenthusiastic when you find something that 'looks' beautiful. Caution is the keyword in mushroom foraging.

Things Needed to Forage and Pick Mushrooms

When you actually go out and start foraging for mushrooms, you need to have the following elements:

A mesh bag or a basket - A good mushroom forager is one who helps in distributing spores to other parts of the forest area. Using a mesh bag, wicker basket, or picnic-style hamper is a great element to take with you. The spores from the mushrooms will fall into the wicker container, and as you walk in the forest area, these spores will fall off and repopulate the forest floor with mushroom seeds.

A brush - A brush is an extremely useful tool to clear the dust from the picked mushrooms before you put them into your basket. The less dirt your bag has, the easier it will be to wash and clean the mushrooms before you cook and eat them.

Another good idea is to attach some **fluorescent tape** to the brush's handles so that you can easily find it if you drop it accidentally in the grass or somewhere on the ground.

A pocket knife - A knife is an essential tool for the following activities:

- To clean the stems of the mushrooms

- To cut the stems to check for worms

- To, sometimes, extract mushrooms cleanly from the ground

Any kitchen knife works well for mushroom foraging, although a foldable pocket knife is best to prevent accidental cuts and bruises from the exposed blade when not in use. Like you did for the brush, make sure you wrap the fluorescent paper around the handle for easy visibility.

Necessary permits - Some government land, especially forest areas, require permits for mushroom foraging activities. Often, these permits are given free of cost for non-commercial use. The permit will state the limit on the number of mushrooms you can pick. For example, your permit could state that you can pick up to 2 gallons of mushrooms per day for 15 days per calendar year.

Also, you might need special permits to forage for special, exotic, or endangered species of mushrooms. For example, foraging for matsutake mushrooms in the Pacific Northwest region requires a special permit to be obtained. The local Forest Service Ranger stations usually provide foragers with maps showing which areas are permissible for foraging.

A pen and notebook - Making notes as you forage through the wild is a great way to learn about mushrooms. Make detailed notes of the location, the tree, stump, or area you picked mushrooms from, and all other relevant details. You could use an audio-recording camera to take videos and/or pictures and record your observations too.

A topographic map - Certain species of mushrooms tend to grow at specific elevations depending on the humidity and temperature at the place and altitude. The internet is likely to give you access to topographic maps. However, access to the internet is likely to be distorted and weak in forest areas. Therefore, it would be a good idea to take along a hard copy of topographic maps of the region in which you are going for mushroom foraging. These hard copies issued by US Forest Services can be freely downloaded in PDF formats.

Something to eat and drink - As you climb up and down mountains and hills, you are highly likely to work up thirst and hunger. It might be a great idea to carry some food and water for your use. Moreover, if in the case of an unlikely but possible scenario wherein you get lost in the wilderness, you might have to wait for a while before a rescue team reaches you. You need food and water to survive in such situations too. Always carry some light snacks and a water bottle while you are on your mushroom foraging trip.

Some desirable elements that could enhance your foraging experience are:

Walkie-talkies - If the mushroom foraging expedition involves a big group of friends or other foragers, then a set of walkie-talkies might be a great idea to communicate with each other. However, for those not wanting to invest too much, a working whistle can work fine too, provided the members of the group are not very far from each other.

Bright clothes - Remember, you are here to forage for mushrooms, not remain inconspicuous, or get lost in the colors of nature. Wear bright-colored clothing to ensure you are easily locatable by the search party in case of the unlikely chance you get lost in the wild. Also, if you are part of a group, then you can remain visible to your forager friends.

An offline GPS device - Considering the internet accessibility in remote forest areas will act up, it might be a good idea to get an offline GPS device to help you stay on course and not get lost in the wilderness. Of course, you can have smartphone apps for this purpose, too, although battery usage might cause concern. If you are planning on making mushroom foraging a long-term hobby, then an offline GPS device is a worthy investment.

Bug-spray - In North America, the season of mushroom foraging (typically springtime) coincides with the season of ticks and mosquitoes. Therefore, a bug-spray is not just handy but an essential item to be packed when you set out on your mushroom foraging trip.

And finally, if you are a lonely forager, then it's okay, go ahead and have your own fun. However, foraging with friends, human and/or canine varieties, can be a lot more fun. The chances of finding great mushrooms automatically increase if you combine the activity with your friends.

Friends can give you second opinions with regard to suspicious-looking mushrooms and species identification. Also, foraging with friends means you have each other's back in case of an unfortunate accident. Moreover, a well-trained and loyal canine can save you from dangerous wildlife as well as some lowlifes who might be lurking to mug you when you are alone.

Don't Waste the Picked Mushrooms - Use Or Preserve Them

More often than not, you are likely to pick far more mushrooms than you actually need in the immediate future. Fresh edible mushrooms are great taste-enhancers when used in soups, pasta, and other dishes. Most of the edible ones are delicious when fried or grilled.

If you cannot use the foraged mushrooms immediately, then the next best thing is to preserve them for future use. The cardinal rules for mushroom preservation are:

- Pick only as many mushrooms as you can reasonably use and/or preserve within a few days of foraging. It would be unwise to pick more mushrooms than you can eat and preserve.

- You should preserve only those mushrooms that are in excellent condition and have been cleaned thoroughly.

- Make sure you label each container of preserved mushrooms with details like the types of mushroom, when they were picked and preserved, where they were found, and other pertinent and interesting information.

There are various ways to preserve mushrooms at home. Another chapter in this book deals in detail about cleaning and preserving foraged mushrooms.

And finally, don't forget that mushroom foraging requires you to be a continuous learner. In addition, give back to the world of mushroom foraging in your own small little way. For example, if you live in an area where mushrooms are found in plenty, then it is quite likely a mushroom foragers' club is active there. Enroll in the club and be an active member of it.

Clubs like these typically have members with varying levels of experience right from a novice forager up to those who have years of experience in foraging mushrooms. The interactions with the members of such clubs will not only help you gain sufficient knowledge from others but also will allow you to share what you know with others as you gradually build your experience in this fascinating field.

Another highly useful aspect of joining such clubs is that they organize foraging expeditions usually headed by experienced foragers. They usually organize informative talks and discussions with other experts in the field, including biologists, chefs, authors, and medical professionals, to spread knowledge about mushroom foraging.

If you do not have access to a real club close to your living area, then you can opt for online forums formed by mushroom foragers. Online versions also offer great opportunities for learning and knowing about mushrooms. You can ask for photos and identification tips from experienced people in the forum. If you know some of the answers, then you get the opportunity to share what you know with others as well.

Whether you choose to join a local club or a virtual online version, remember that maintaining a symbiotic relationship is the best way for optimal outcomes for you as well as the club. A small word of caution here.

While experienced foragers are quite happy to share their knowledge expertise with you, especially about wrong choices of mushrooms and how to distinguish between edible and poisonous ones, many foragers are quite guarded about sharing information regarding their favorite foraging grounds. And this hesitant attitude is perfectly understandable, considering that it can take years to find lucrative spaces that have an abundance of your favorite mushrooms.

Therefore, don't be offended if experienced foragers don't divulge details of their favorite mushroom foraging spots. But nearly all enthusiasts are happy to share details like the general layout of a particular area, the ideal elevation where specific mushrooms can be found easily, details about indicator plants around which certain types of mushrooms tend to grow, etc. After this, it is up to you to explore the region and find your own great hunting spots. And moreover, this exploration is the primary fun aspect of mushroom foraging.

Therefore, take help and then do your own thing. With patience and a bit of dedication, you will move from a novice to an experienced forager sooner than later. This book deals in detail with a few important and common mushrooms found in North America. You will find a lot more information about the following mushrooms in the next few chapters:

- Morels

- Chanterelles

- Fairy Ring Mushrooms

- Sweet Tooth Mushrooms

- Meadow Mushrooms

- Shaggy Mane Mushrooms

- Hen of the Wood

- Bear's Head Tooth Mushrooms

- Giant Puffballs

- Chaga Mushrooms

- Reishi Mushrooms

- Sulfur Shelf Mushrooms

- Black Trumpet Mushrooms

This book has a few chapters dedicated to these mushrooms, explaining the identifying characteristics, how to discern an edible variety from a toxic look-alike, and a couple of easy recipes to cook certain special varieties of mushrooms. So, read on and build your knowledge levels before you start off on your mushroom exploration trips.

Chapter Three

Cleaning and Preserving Mushrooms

There is little doubt that foraging is one of the most fun and magical hobbies to follow. It's fun to think of exploring unknown territories, discovering exotic mushrooms, having your wicker basket overflowing with mushrooms, returning home to look at your collection with awe and happiness. It's exciting cooking and eating the delicious dishes, sharing them with your friends and family, and everything related to mushroom foraging.

After you finish everything listed above, you look at your basket and realize you still have so many mushrooms left, and now you are stumped. What to do with such a big collection? Wasting them is not an option because it is not the behavior of an ethical mushroom forager.

Well, preserving is a great option because you can keep your collected mushrooms for a longer time and use them as additions to multiple dishes. In fact, preserving foraged mushrooms is a bounteous thing to do for all mushroom foragers. The process of preserving mushrooms starts with cleaning them.

How to Clean Mushrooms

Cleaning mushrooms can be quite a chore considering that many varieties, especially the popular ones like chanterelles, carry a lot of litter from the forest floor. Here are some tips on cleaning mushrooms with water:

Put a few of them (do them in small batches) into a colander with small perforations. Run them under tap water directly from the faucet. Use a small brush to remove the dirt from the mushrooms even as they are being washed by running water. Once your mushrooms are cleaned thoroughly, put them in a bigger colander with larger perforations for draining.

Once the mushrooms are completely drained of water, spread them on a single towel and leave them overnight to ensure all the moisture is removed and they are totally dried. Use the following tips to clean mushrooms before cooking them:

1. Before you rinse your mushroom, slice them to your desired size. Halve, quarter, or slice your mushrooms before you clean them in water so that you get more surface area resulting in cleaner mushrooms than if you tried to rinse them wholly without cutting.

2. Place the mushrooms inside a colander and space them out so that each of the pieces gets ample exposure to water for rinsing.

3. Small varieties like the button mushrooms just need a quick rinse to remove all dirt.

4. Ensure the faucet is running at medium pressure, and the water is at room temperature.

5. Then, dry off the rinsed mushrooms and examine each piece thoroughly and cut off those parts from where dirt or mold could not be removed by rinsing.

6. For mushrooms that should not be water-rinsed, you can use a damp paper towel to rub off any caked-on sediments. Alternatively, you can use a fresh toothbrush dipped in a bit of water to do so.

Different Methods of Preserving Mushrooms

Some of the common ways of preserving mushrooms include:

- Drying

- Freezing

- Powdering

- Tincturing

- Pickling

- Making mushroom ketchup

Let us look at each of them in a bit of detail:

Drying Mushrooms

When you thoroughly dry mushrooms, you can keep them for a longer time than fresh ones. For example, if you end up with a lot of mushrooms when you go foraging during fall, then you can simply dry them up. In the dried state, you can use them right through the winter months as well. There are various methods of drying mushrooms:

- Lay them out in the sun after cleaning them thoroughly.

- Place them in a dehydrator overnight at a temperature of around 115 to 120 degrees F. By morning, the mushrooms will become a little crispy like fries.

Use these tips for drying your mushrooms (typically you will get 1.5 ounces of dried mushrooms from one pound of fresh ones):

- Slice the mushrooms thinly. The slices should not be more than ½-inch in thickness. The thumb rule is this. The thicker the flesh, the thinner should be your slice. Then, you can dry them out in the sun using any of these methods:

- String the sliced mushrooms and hang them to dry in an airy room, which gets a lot of sunlight. Alternately, you can put them out into direct sunlight, especially when the weather is warm.

- You can spread out the slices on a wire screen, which can be placed on a heat register for the mushrooms to dry slowly.

- The trick is to dry mushrooms until they break like a cracker. If the mushroom only bends or still seems moist, then you must continue the drying process until it becomes 'cracker dry.'

- Simply lay them in a single layer on a sheet newspaper and put them out to dry. You would need to repeat this process every day, turning the sliced mushrooms over occasionally until they are completely dry. It is important not to crowd the mushrooms.

It is better not to dry mushrooms in an oven because it requires a lot of continuous monitoring. If you let them dry in an oven unchecked for very long, then your mushrooms can become extremely hard and inedible as it gets very difficult to rehydrate them. You can store the completely dried mushrooms in an airtight container with a small packet of desiccant to prevent moisture absorption in the future as well. Attach a label on the container with the following details:

- Type of mushroom

- Date collected

- Place collected

- Date preserved

- Any other important information

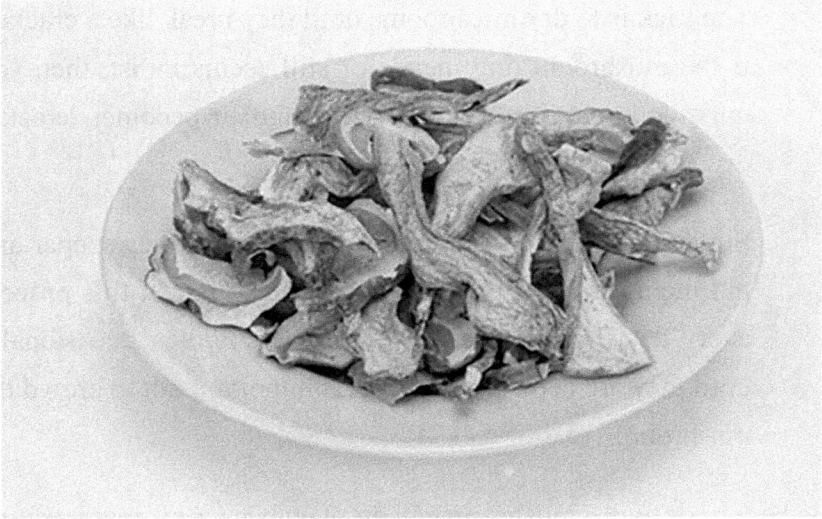

Next, freeze them airtight container for a week to ensure any microbes that might have made their way into the mushrooms during the dehydration process. After a week of freezing it, remove the container and store it in a dry place.

You can also use a food hydrator to dry and preserve mushrooms. Arrange the sliced mushrooms on the racks of the food hydrator, ensuring they are not overcrowded. Slow drying at a lower temperature (about 150 degrees C) over a longer period is better than quickly drying at high temperatures. Higher temperatures tend to damage mushrooms and their nutrients.

The process for rehydrating these dried mushrooms is very simple. Soak them in warm water for about 15-20 minutes, and your mushrooms are ready for use. Also, don't discard the water in which the mushrooms were soaked because it will absorb the flavors of the dried mushrooms. Therefore, you can use it in cooking your dishes. It would be like a mushroom stock.

You can use the drying method for morels, Shiitake, etc. Black trumpet mushrooms (found abundantly in the northeastern parts of North America) are one of the best varieties of mushrooms to be used in the dried form. They get a smoky, aromatic, and pleasantly fruity flavor when they are dry. They can be harvested during summer and used in the dry form right through winter.

The advantage of drying mushrooms include:

- Drying is the best method to preserve the flavor for a very long time. In fact, drying intensifies the flavor of many mushroom species.

- It is very easy and convenient to store dried mushrooms. There is no need for any special equipment.

The disadvantages of drying mushrooms are:

- Drying is likely to change the texture of mushrooms, making them quite tough.

- Aromas are often lost in the drying process.

- Rehydration does not restore the texture of mushrooms to earlier levels.

- Using dehydrating machines can be expensive and elaborate.

Freezing Mushrooms

Button mushrooms are great to preserve through freezing methods. You can leave the small-sized button mushrooms as they are, and slice the larger ones. The mushrooms for freezing must not be longer than about 1 inch. You can use any one of the following methods to freeze mushrooms:

- Sauté them in a little bit of butter or olive oil. Then cool them to room temperature and then transfer the mushrooms to plastic containers or freezer bags.

- You can steam the mushrooms over boiling water or a steaming pot. After about 10 minutes of steaming, cool your mushrooms, and transfer them to containers or bags.

- You can also blanch the mushrooms before freezing them. Whichever method you use to cook your mushrooms for not more than 10 minutes, you must cool them completely before transferring them to freezer packs or plastic containers.

The label of the container must have more detail than just that it's dried mushrooms. That information is details of whether the mushrooms were sautéed, blanched, or steamed and the date of the cooking process. Matsutake, Verpa, morels, pig's ears, and chanterelles are great to preserve by the freezing method.

The advantages of blanching and freezing partially cooked mushrooms as a preserving method are:

- Blanching is a great way to clean the mushrooms as well as prevent them from becoming mushy.

- Dirt and sand are all removed through blanching without affecting the flavors of the frozen end product.

- This preservation process is convenient for large quantities in a short period.

- You can just put frozen mushrooms into your soups as pre-thawing is not necessary.

One of the biggest disadvantages of blanching and freezing is that the frozen mushrooms are not suitable for frying, sautéing, or any form of crisping of mushrooms.

The advantages of steaming and freezing mushrooms include:

- Steaming is quite convenient.

- The end frozen product is more versatile than the blanched and frozen end product.

- The texture and flavors are excellently preserved.

The disadvantages of the steaming and freezing method are:

- Steaming takes more time and effort than the blanching process.

- Dirt and sand are not removed as well as in the blanching process. Therefore, you must select only those mushrooms that are thoroughly cleaned for this process. You should use other freezing methods for others.

The advantages of sautéing and freezing method of mushroom preservation are:

- Convenient and easy, the texture and taste of the mushrooms preserved in this way are the best of the three.

- The quality of texture and flavor is not retained for as long as the other two methods.

Pickling Mushrooms

For pickling mushrooms, you will need some extra ingredients. Also, mason jars with bands and lids work best for storing your pickled mushrooms. It is a done thing that you sterilize the jars before storing your pickled mushrooms. Here is a simple method to sterilize mason jars:

- Put the jar in boiling water for about 10 minutes.

- Then, remove the jar from the hot water with a pair of tongs, and place it on a clean towel to dry.

Other ingredients needed for pickling mushrooms are (the given measurements are good for six cups of mushrooms):

10 Peppercorns

Sprigs of thyme

Dried hot chili

Garlic cloves

Kosher salt

White vinegar

Olive oil

Granulated sugar

Clean the mushrooms well. Using a variety of mushrooms is a great way to make the pickle highly flavorful. Boil the mushrooms for a little more time than you would in case of drying or freezing the mushrooms. About 15 minutes would do.

Bring to boil all the other ingredients mentioned above in water so that you can get a nicely-spiced sauce. When this sauce is nicely boiled, pour it over the cooked mushrooms. Fill the sterilized jars with the pickled mushrooms and pour some more sauce until the mushrooms are fully covered.

Seal the lid on the filled mason jar and allow it to cool to room temperature, after which you must refrigerate the pickled mushrooms. You can use a variety of spices and herbs to pickle your mushrooms depending on your likes/dislikes and how each spice marries with each mushroom.

The advantages of pickling mushrooms are:

- Pickle broths used to marinate mushrooms intensify the flavors. Therefore, pickling is excellent to preserve bland varieties.

- It is relatively easy to pickle mushrooms at home.

- The disadvantages of the pickling method are:

- You require proven recipes, and it is imperative that you strictly adhere to the recipes.

- It is not a great method to experiment because wrong pickling can result in food poisoning.

Preserving the extra harvested mushrooms is good not only for you but also a reflection of your respect for the fruits of nature. By preserving picked mushrooms, you are essentially telling Mother Nature that you value every little thing she gives you. Therefore, make sure you don't pick more than you need, and if you do, for some reason, ensure nothing is wasted.

Chapter Four

Morels and Chanterelles

The next few chapters are focused on particular wild mushrooms that can be foraged in North America. We start with the common favorites, namely morels and chanterelles.

Morels

Morel mushrooms are found abundantly across North America, especially the United States growing under hardwood trees. The harvest season for morels consists of a very short window during springtime. This harvest window varies from place to place. Distinctive features of morel mushrooms include:

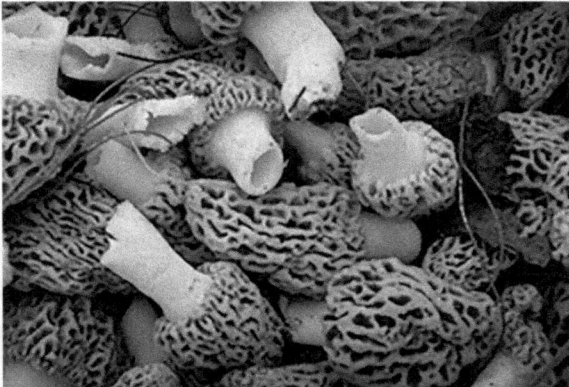

The yellowish-gray and deeply wrinkled 'honeycombed' cap, which is hollow through the center. This mushroom is typically 2 to 9 cm in height and 2 to 5 cm in thickness. Some poisonous varieties have honeycombed caps like the edible morels. When in doubt, keep them in a separate container to check with experts later on or don't pick them at all.

Morels have a very strong taste and are at their delicious best when cooked with butter. Morels with leeks are a favorite combination for many mushroom lovers.

There are many questions which you have to pay attention to while looking for morel mushrooms. Questions such as when to look, where to look, what they look like, what looks like them, and more.

When to look: It is important to know that the best time to harvest morel mushrooms is during springtime. Black morels are the first ones to arrive, and they are followed by yellow morels about three weeks later. Morels have also been spotted during winter. They really have a mind of their own when it comes to when they want to grow.

Where to look: Morel mushrooms occupy the temperate zones of both hemispheres. Unlike some mushrooms, morels do not grow on trees. They do not grow on wood. You will always find them on the ground, growing in groups or in clusters. Sometimes they are just scattered, and some are even found growing all alone. If you come across one morel, stop and look around. Chances are you will find many more within the vicinity. Take a look around areas that are covered by the tree shadows, and you are bound to come across a cluster or two.

It is easier to locate the type of morels mushrooms if you know which tree they ground around. Most morels are associated with their own tree around which they grow.

Since black morels are the first ones to appear during morel season, we will talk about them first. They generally grow around coniferous trees and are mostly found in north-western America. Areas with human activity are also favorable for the growth of morel mushrooms. Black morels are also found near ash, so visiting burnt areas would make finding morels very easy.

Yellow morels are more common in eastern North America and in the Midwestern countries. They grow around hardwood trees, including tulip, ash, poplar, and dead or dying elm trees. They also grow in old apple orchards.

These are just general places where you might find what you are looking for. There are instances where yellow morels grow around coniferous trees, and black morels grow around hardwood trees.

Study shows that morels love to grow in alkaline soils. This explains their preference for apple orchards and burnt areas. Forest fires create ash, which boosts the alkalinity of the surrounding soil. Apple trees also favor alkaline soils for growth. So before planting apple trees, the soil is treated with calcium carbonate, which is a process called liming. The new, treated, alkaline soil proves to be a favorable condition for the growth of morels.

What they look like: many species of mushrooms can be categorized into black and yellow morels. Morels take on a conical shape. They are long and lean mushrooms, unlike most common mushrooms, which are short and wide. Morels take on a variety of colors. The caps have characteristic dull colors like yellow-brown, gray, grayish-black, olive, etc, while the stalk takes on a whitish color. The caps of morel mushrooms are very different from other mushrooms. Once you know what to look for, it will be hard to misidentify a morel mushroom.

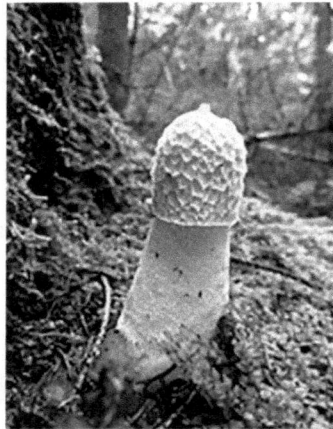

Their caps are ridged on the outside, and they have a honeycomb-like appearance inside. Their caps are also fully attached to the stalk. It seems as if the caps emerge from the stalk and meet at the top. When we cut open a morel mushroom lengthwise, we can see that it is filled with a cottony substance.

What looks like them: There are many toxic look-alikes of morels, and it is important to learn to discern between them so that you don't end up consuming the wrong ones. Yet, the differences between them are not very difficult to learn and master although as a novice, you must take second opinions in case of doubt (keep them in a separate basket to ask an expert later on, or someone in your group can help too), or better still, don't pick them up until you are absolutely sure.

- **Half - free morels**: this mushroom isn't exactly a look-alike of a morel mushroom except for the fact that it has a white stalk. The caps of the half-free morels are short. Moreover, when we cut open this mushroom lengthwise, we can see that the cap does not originate fully from the stalk, rather it is only half attached to the stalk. Hence the name half-free morels.

- **Wrinkled thimble-cap**: as the name suggests, this mushroom has a very wrinkled cap, unlike a morel mushroom, which has a ridged cap. These mushrooms are very short. Their cap is attached to the tip of the stalk and spreads in all directions from the tip like an umbrella. The sides of the cap hang freely.

- **False morels**: the differences between false and true morels are as clear as night and day. False morels are short mushrooms with a wrinkled, dark reddish colored cap. Their stock is very wide as well. When you cut lengthwise, false morels appear folded on the inside, whereas true morels appear hollow with a cottony filling. It is important to differentiate between false and true morels. Some species of false morels like G.esculenta, on consumption, can lead to problems including nausea, fever and fatigue, liver and kidney failure, and sometimes even death.

How to consume: Black and yellow morels are one of the most favored edible mushrooms. But just like all wild mushrooms, it is never meant to be eaten raw. Morels taste best when cooked in butter or oil.

Chanterelles

With more than 15 different species, Chanterelles are another common variety of wild mushrooms found abundantly across North America. They are also available in plenty in Central America, Africa, and Eurasia. Chanterelles typically grow in coniferous forests. But you can also find them in certain specific species in grasslands and in particular locations in mountainous birch and beech forests.

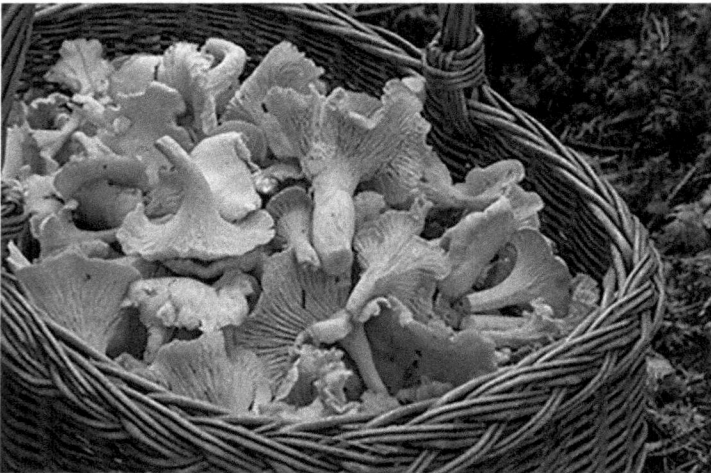

These mushrooms usually grow in clumps among the moss. The harvest season for chanterelles starts from late summer and extends up to December, depending on the location and the species. The distinctive characteristics of chanterelles include:

- Funnel-shaped golden or yellow meaty mushrooms.

- The gill-like ridges under the cap run right along the stem downwards.

- Chanterelles have an earthy, fruity, or woody smell.

Chanterelles have a peppery taste and being quite rich in flavor, turn out excellent dishes that use wines, butter, or cream. Poisonous look-alikes of chanterelles or false chanterelles are darker yellow (almost orange) cap. The caps also have dark centers that fade progressively towards the edges. False chanterelles are rarely fatal. However, they have horrible taste and can also cause stomach problems. Examples of false morels include jack-o-lantern mushrooms.

The ideal weather for the growth of chanterelle mushrooms involves hot and humid days. The days after heavy rains are also very favorable for their growth. Chanterelles take on a reddish-orange color. They are small, but due to their bright color, they are not hard to spot. A very wide range of mushroom species can be categorized as chanterelle mushrooms. In the United States, there are three distinct color groups of chanterelles that are very common.

Red chanterelles: these small and thin-fleshed mushrooms sure are a treat for the eyes. They are also called cinnabars. Cinnabars taste like mild notes of apricots mixed with almonds.

Black chanterelles: often referred to as 'black trumpets,' these mushrooms are larger than cinnabars but smaller than orange chanterelles. They, too, are thin-fleshed. Black trumpets are known for their delicious taste. Typically, they are dried and powdered and cooked in olive oil to create black trumpet oil. This oil is mostly enjoyed with bread.

Orange chanterelles: the orange chanterelles, unlike its name, come in a range of colors including pink, peach, yellow, and of course, orange. Orange chanterelles have a wide variety of sub-species under them with slightly different shapes, colors, and sizes. In the United States, there are hundreds of closely related, yet genetically distinct subspecies of orange chanterelles.

Like black chanterelles, orange chanterelles are also delicious when cooked. They have a subtle taste with hints of apricots and almonds.

Where to find orange chanterelle mushrooms: these mushrooms are found abundantly in the United States. In fact, it is found in all the states except Hawaii as the weather conditions of Hawaii aren't favorable for their growth.

They form a symbiotic relationship with their surrounding trees. This means their host tree feeds them, and they feed their host trees. This is why chanterelles are often found growing in mature and thick forests. They are prominently found around oak, beech, and maple, and sometimes, even evergreen trees.

When chanterelles grow: these mushrooms love hot and humid conditions. Heavy rain will start the growth of chanterelle mushrooms, and within two weeks of rain, you will find prominent growth of chanterelle mushrooms.

What chanterelles look like: the most prominent species of chanterelle mushrooms are the red, black, and orange species. It is very easy to find orange chanterelles because of their abundance and large size. Apart from their colors, almost all chanterelles take on a vase-like shape. The underside of these mushrooms consists of false gills. These false gills fork, unlike true gills that are individual blades. They are found to grow either alone or in small clusters near trees. They give out a very sweet and fruity smell.

It is important to know about their poisonous look-alikes as well. Here are some important look-alikes:

- **Jack-o-lantern mushrooms**: these mushrooms are poisonous. They have a characteristic bright orange color, and their gills have a green glow at night. They grow around dead and decaying trees, and they are mostly found in clusters.

- **False chanterelles**: these mushrooms look very similar to the true chanterelles. It is safe to consume these mushrooms, but some people have reported no side effects despite having consumed these mushrooms, and others have complained of stomach aches and fever. It is best to stay away from these mushrooms. Unlike true chanterelles, these mushrooms have true gills in the underside layer of their cap.

- **Hedgehog mushrooms**: if you come across this mushroom, you consume it without any second thoughts. They taste delicious. The catch is that they are much rarer than orange chanterelles. You know you have found hedgehog mushrooms if you see tiny white teeth in the cap's underside. This is where the spores are released.

How to Harvest Chanterelles

Once you have identified chanterelles, it is time to harvest them.

1. Cut the mushrooms at the base of the stem so as not to harm the neighboring clusters and reduce the time you need to clean your mushrooms.

2. Make sure to pick only clean chanterelles and leave behind the ones covered in mud. Plus, the ones you leave behind will give out spores that will grow into fresh chanterelles.

3. It's best to harvest the old and large ones rather than the young and small ones. This ensures that they have produced spores already.

4. Use a filter or a breathable basket while carrying chanterelles so that they give out spores over the areas they are being carried to. This gives birth to new chanterelle colonies.

5. Do not pluck chanterelles and store them for later use. They will start to go bad within two days. If you keep them refrigerated, they can live up to a week or two.

How to Cook Them

• The first step is to dehydrate them and powder them. Chanterelles are 95% water, which can later be used to add flavor to other dishes.

• Sauté them in butter or oil for twenty minutes. Let them cool and put them in Ziplock bags in the fridge. This method takes up more storage space than dehydrated mushrooms, but the flavor stays in the mushroom for a longer period.

Morels and chanterelles are found abundantly in North America, and even as a novice mushroom forager, you are unlikely to miss them when you are on your hunt.

Chapter Five

Fairy Ring Mushrooms
and Sweet Tooth Mushrooms

Fairy Ring Mushrooms

Marasmius oreades is commonly referred to as fairy ring mushrooms. The unique name 'fairy ring mushrooms' comes from old folklore. It was believed that these mushrooms which grow in circles follow the path laid by fairies dancing in a circle or a ring. And if you stepped into the ring, you might be compelled to join in the dance. Widely distributed across North America, fairy ring mushrooms usually grow in grassy areas like fields, lawns, and dunes.

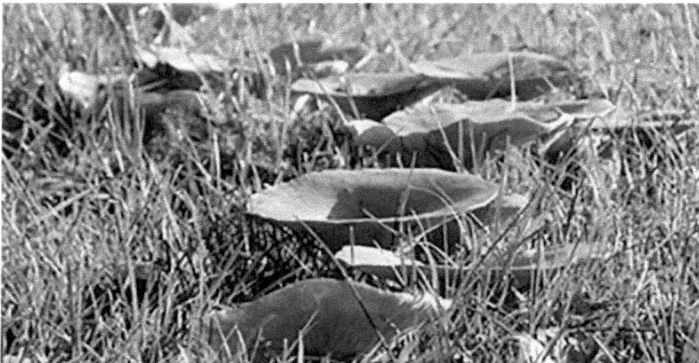

You can also find them in craters formed by dead tree stumps. They can be harvested in summer as well as in fall. In warm climates, fairy ring mushrooms can be harvested right through the year.

Distinctive features of fairy ring mushrooms include:

- They grow in an arc or a ring.

- Their caps are usually 1 to 5 cm in diameter.

- At an immature stage, their caps are sometimes rolled inwards. However, as the mushrooms mature, the caps become upturned.

- Sometimes, the caps of fairy ring mushrooms are described as nipple-like because of a prominent center.

- The gills are widely spaced, and some are forked, which means they are not entirely connected with the stem.

- The color of fairy ring mushrooms is a usually pale buff or tan, and sometimes white too. They are dry and bald.

- A highly reliable characteristic of fairy ring mushrooms is that the stem is very tough and pliable.

The stems have to be separated from the cap as they cannot be cooked. The intact caps require to be rinsed with cold water and then allowed to dry. As they don't have a very strong taste, you can add your favorite spices to make them as delicious as you want.

Fairy Ring Mushrooms are found in sunny and open areas. You can find them in grassy meadows, yards, and pastures. As these mushrooms grow, the mycelium uses up all the nutrients from the soil resulting in the grass on which these mushrooms grow to dry up. This is the reason you tend to see a ring of dry grass around the edge of the mycelium.

When the central mycelium uses up all the nutrients from the surrounding soil, it dies, resulting in all the nutrients being returned to the soil. Consequently, the grass begins to grow again, forming a ring of fresh grass over the earlier dried ring.

A few more important characteristics of the stem of fairy ring mushrooms are:

- The stem is tough and pliable, which means you can bend the stem back and forth, but it will not break.

- It is important to take care while you cut the stem before cooking because the cap might tear if you use too much pressure.

- One of the features that help you distinguish fairy ring mushrooms from others is the stem quality. The stems of other mushrooms break easily.

Cooking with fairy ring mushrooms - First, you must gently cut off the stem from the cap. The cap has to be in one piece after it is separated from the stem. The best way to keep the cap intact is by gently twisting the stem, which will pop off the cap. Fairy ring mushrooms are quite easy to clean, considering that not much dirt is found on them. You can do a quick rinse to remove all the dirt from the caps.

Preserving fairy ring mushrooms is very easy too. They are so light that drying them in the sun is the simplest method. An important point to note here is that fairy ring mushrooms can dry quite quickly, and therefore, you must check on them regularly to prevent them from shriveling excessively. Also, if there are signs of impending rain, then make sure you bring in the drying mushrooms because, with just a little bit of moisture, they can be rehydrated.

Nutritional benefits - Thanks to the very small-sized edible caps, fairy ring mushrooms are rarely used as the main component of any dish. They are primarily used to flavor dishes (they have a sweetish, almost cinnamon-like taste) and to give the texture of the dish an interesting twist. They are very healthy mushrooms considering their high protein and fiber content and low fat and carb content.

A toxic look-alike is the deadly Fool's Funnel that has potentially fatal levels of muscarine, a dangerous toxin. Another problem with fairy ring mushrooms is that since they grow in grasslands and lawns, the toxic effects of pesticides that are often sprayed could be absorbed by the mushrooms. Therefore, if you find fairy ring mushrooms in your foraging expedition, then you must understand the status of the grassland or meadow you have picked them from.

Fairy Ring Mushroom Sauce Pasta

Ingredients:

- Fairy ring mushrooms (cleaned) - 2 ounces

- Capellini pasta - 4 ounces (you can use any pasta of your choice)

- Diced shallots - 1 tbsp

- Unsalted butter - 3 tbsp

- Dry white wine - ⅛ cup

- Chicken stock - ½ cup (you can use any poultry stock or even vegetable stock if you wish to go vegan with this dish)

Directions:

Cook the pasta in salted boiling water until al dente. In another pan, melt 2 tbsp of butter and fry them for a few minutes until they are brown. Season with salt and pepper. Add the wine and cook for a couple of minutes more. Then add the chicken, poultry, or vegetable stock and bring the mixture to a boil.

Add the al dente pasta and stir continuously. Add the remaining butter. Stir to get a great pasta dish in a creamy sauce.

Sweet Tooth Mushrooms

Also known as a **wood hedgehog** or **hedgehog mushrooms**, sweet tooth mushrooms are widely distributed across North America, Australia, Europe, and northern parts of Asia. In North America, sweet tooth mushrooms fruit around white oak trees, and in the northern parts of the continent, they grow around pine trees.

Their harvest seasons start from around mid-summer and continue into late fall. One of the best things about sweet tooth mushrooms is that bugs are not attracted to them, which is a refreshing change from other varieties of mushrooms wherein many of the good ones get rapidly infested by bugs, especially during summer.

The sweet tooth hedgehog mushrooms have teeth or spine-like structures instead of gills under their caps. These teeth are the defining feature of this mushroom variety. Other features include:

- The caps look similar to those of chanterelle mushrooms, although this variety has a darker, almost orangish tan, rather than the golden-yellow of chanterelles.

- The sweet tooth mushroom bruises to a yellowish-brown or dark orange color.

- The caps are mostly broadly convex in shape, although they do come in other shapes too. The diameter of the caps varies between 2 to 17 cm.

- The gills range from a whitish to a light-brown color and are tooth-like in structure.

- The stem of the sweet tooth mushrooms are usually off-centered and are often irregularly shaped.

There are not many common poisonous look-alikes. The sweet tooth mushroom has a sweet, nutty flavor, are crunchy and can also be frozen. Two closely related species represent sweet tooth mushrooms, namely Hydnum repandum and Hydnum umbilicatum.

Some basic differences between these two species include:

- The cap of Hydnum repandum varies between 2 and 8 inches in diameter. It is thick and mostly convex, though caps of other shapes also are seen. They get an orangish color when bruised. The cap of Hydnum umbilicatum is generally smaller and has a sunken depression at the top. The stem of this species is more centered than the Hydnum repandum.

- The flesh of Hydnum repandum is whitish, thick, and stains to an orangish color when brushed. The flesh of Hydnum umbilicatum is thin and whitish but does not stain when bruised.

- Hydnum umbilicatum can be found in wet areas and under conifers from around August until November though they are more prominently seen in September and October. If you find one Hydnum umbilicatum, you are likely to find many more in the vicinity. Hydnum repandum can be found near hardwood trees like birch and beech.

Sweet tooth mushrooms taste delicious when they are simply sautéed or fried in butter. You can also dry them to preserve them. They have a crunchy texture, and their smell and flavor are both quite similar to chanterelles. The smell of sweet tooth mushrooms intensifies when they are dried. Some mushroom experts believe that hedgehog mushrooms are under-appreciated because of the more widely available and popular chanterelles.

Cleaning sweet tooth mushrooms can be quite tricky because grains of sand can get stuck in the wide gaps between the teeth. It would be best for you first to brush off all the visible grit and grime, and then give a quick rinse under running tap water to make sure all the dirt is removed. It is important not to keep them for very long in water because they tend to become waterlogged. After a quick rinse, keep them in a paper towel to dry. If your mushrooms are relatively clean, then simply brushing them with a pastry brush will do the trick.

Pickling sweet tooth mushrooms is a great way to preserve them. Drying them may not be a great idea because, like chanterelles, the texture and flavor changes after they are rehydrated and become something quite different from the original state.

Potato Hash with Sweet Tooth Mushrooms

Ingredients:

- Olive oil - 4 tbsp

- Shallots (diced) - 4 (if you are using onion, then one medium-sized would be enough)

- Medium potatoes (cubed) - 2-4

- Celery (chopped) - 1 cup

- Fresh thyme - a few sprigs

- Sweet tooth mushrooms (chopped) - 2-3 cups

- Chives - 3-5 leaves (you can use garlic chives for added flavor)

Directions:

Sauté the onions or shallots using 3 tbsp of oil until they are soft and translucent. Toss the potatoes and cook for about 20 minutes until the cubes of potatoes are cooked enough for you to be able to pierce a fork through them. Now, add the chives, celery, and thyme and continue to cook until the celery is done, stirring occasionally. Remove this from the heat and keep aside in a bowl.

Now, cook the sweet tooth mushrooms in the remaining tablespoon of oil for about 5-10 minutes until the mushrooms get soft. Add the potato hash back into the pan and mix thoroughly. Serve hot.

Chapter Six

Meadow Mushrooms and Shaggy Mane Mushrooms

Meadow Mushrooms

The good news for beginners is that meadow mushrooms (Agaricus campestris) need not really be 'foraged' because they can be seen in plenty lying around randomly. They usually start fruiting from early summer. When you find meadow mushrooms, you are likely to find a bunch of them together. And even better is when you find such a place, then store the location somewhere because if you return the next year around the same time, you will definitely find it growing repeatedly in the same area.

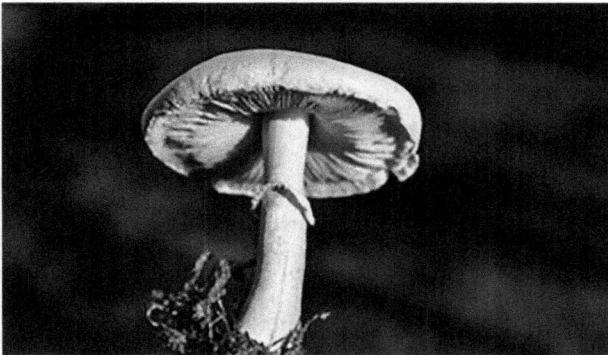

Meadow mushrooms are also called field mushrooms and are found across North America. They also grow abundantly in Asia, Europe, New Zealand, and North Africa. Generally found in grasslands, meadow mushrooms can grow in the form of a ring (like fairy ring mushrooms) or as a standalone variety. They are commonly found in California's Great Central Valley. Meadow mushrooms can be harvested in summer, spring, and in fall after the rains. Identifying characteristics include:

- A white cap with a diameter ranging between 5 to 10 cm.

- The cap is flat when the mushroom is mature.

- The gills under the cap are pink in color during the immature stage, and as the mushrooms mature, these gills turn to reddish-brown in the juvenile stage, and finally to dark brown when it is completely mature.

- The stalk, stem, or stipe of meadow mushrooms range between 3 to 10 cm in height.

- The spore is reddish-brown.

- Meadow mushrooms bruise to a reddish-brown color.

There are many fatal look-alike species, and therefore, it is imperative that if you discard all similar-looking mushrooms that don't have the pinkish gills. Amanita virosa (with white gills) is a deadly mushroom that closely resembles the meadow mushroom. Another dangerous look-alike is Amanita ocreata, which has a white cap and white to pinkish color fruiting bodies. A separate chapter in this book deals with poisonous mushrooms.

Meadow mushrooms are similar in taste to button mushrooms, although with a shorter shelf life. Field mushrooms can be fried or sautéed or even eaten raw, and therefore, are often added to salads. Meadow mushrooms are well-preserved by freezing (after duly steaming, blanching, or sautéing) or pickling them. Dried meadow mushrooms can be powdered and used in broths and soups and also as seasonings.

A few look-alikes of meadow mushrooms do exist, especially ones with similar pink gills. Here are some tips to correctly identify the edible meadow mushrooms and not pick the toxic (although they are not known to be fatal) ones:

- Cut the stem of the mushroom you have picked in the hope that they are meadow mushrooms. Wait for about 15 minutes. If the stem stains yellow, then what you have picked is not the edible meadow mushroom. Throw it away.

- Smell the underside of the caps. If you get a pleasant 'mushroomy' odor, then you are good to go. If you get an unpleasant smell, then throw it away.

- Meadow mushrooms have a distinctive ring right around the middle of the stem.

- Meadow mushrooms have some excellent medicinal and cosmetic benefits, including:

- Extracts of this meadow are used in cosmetics for their skin conditioning properties.

- They are used as a bioindicator to trace silver concentrations in any medium.

- Environmentalist experts believe that meadow mushrooms can be useful in decontaminating soil, which has been exposed to engine oils.

- Therapeutic benefits of meadow mushrooms include a blood-glucose regulator, an antioxidant, an antimicrobial, etc.

- Meadow mushrooms have a good concentration of linoleic acid, an essential fatty acid in the human diet.

Provencal Meadow Mushrooms

Ingredients:

- Meadow mushrooms - 1 pound
- Onion (minced) - ½ cup
- Olive oil - 2 tbsp
- Garlic cloves (minced) - 3
- Parsley (chopped) - ¼ cup
- Lemon juice - for flavoring
- Salt and pepper - to taste

Directions:

Slice the cleaned and wiped mushrooms in thick slices. Place the slices in a large pan over the heat. Soon, the mushrooms will start to sizzle. Soon, the water from them would be released into the pan. At this point, add salt and the minced onions. Very few mushrooms and onions will be swimming in the water from the mushroom. Let this mixture boil until most of the water evaporates.

Now, add the olive oil and toss around to make sure everything in the pan is coated with the oil. Sauté the mixture until it starts to brown. Add garlic and pepper and cook for another minute or two. Finally, add the parsley and toss everything together. Add the lemon juice after removing from the heat and serve hot.

Shaggy Mane Mushrooms

Also referred to as **Shaggy Inkcap**, **Lawyer's Wig**, or **Maned Agaric**, shaggy mane mushrooms (Coprinus comatus) are found in meadows and grasslands all over Europe and North America. They appear straight from out of the ground and can be found in rocky soil, wood chip piles, lawns, or any patch of degraded and compacted land, which makes them an easy hunt for urban foragers.

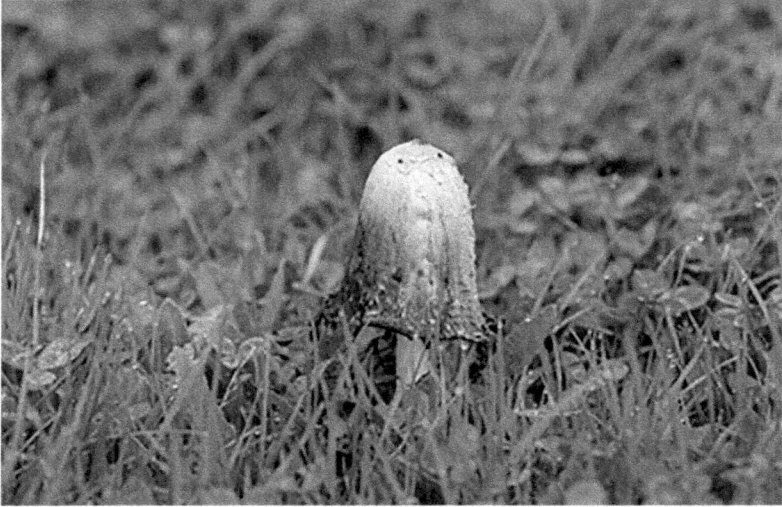

They can be harvested between June and November, depending on the temperature of the place. Picking out shaggy mane mushrooms is quite easy, except for confusing them with ink-cap mushrooms, their toxic twins. In fact, shaggy mane mushrooms are one of the "foolproof four" of easily identifiable mushrooms. The other three are giant puffballs, morels, and chicken of the woods. Identifying characteristics of shaggy mane mushrooms include:

- They are edible only in the immature stage, which means if before the gills turn black in color.

- Spores of shaggy mane mushrooms are of deep black color.

- True to its name, this mushroom has a shaggy cap that droops over and covers almost the entire length of the stem, especially in the immature stage. The shaggy cap has a scaly covering.

- The stem of shaggy mane mushrooms is hollow and fibrous. They are wide at the bottom and taper slowly towards the top, where they are attached to the cap that droops over the stem.

- The gills are white in the mature stage and quickly turn to pink and then to black as the mushroom matures. These mushrooms must be harvested before the gills turn black.

The common toxic look-alikes of shaggy mane mushrooms are the common **ink-cap mushroom**, which can induce nausea, vomiting, and diarrhea, especially when consumed with alcohol. Interestingly, the side-effects of eating ink-cap mushrooms are directly proportional to the amount of alcohol consumed. Some of the common differences between ink-cap and shaggy mane mushrooms are:

- Shaggy manes are taller and stronger than ink-cap mushrooms.

- Shaggy manes commonly grow in singles as against ink-caps, which grow mostly in dense clusters.

- Shaggy manes typically grow from hard ground like packed soil at the edge of a walking or driving trail. Ink-caps usually grow directly from wood.

- Shaggy manes, like their name, are extremely shaggy-looking, making them look like they are wearing wigs. Ink-caps do not have such a shaggy appearance.

The flavor of these mushrooms is almost like something out of a fairy tale eatery. Shaggy mane mushrooms have a lot of water content, and therefore, make excellent soups and stocks. They are also excellent additions in risotto.

However, cooking shaggy manes is not an easy task. The primary problem is that they have a very short shelf life because they are very delicate and tend to damage rapidly. If they are bruised even slightly or just once or twice, they begin to get soft, wet, and dark and quickly turn into an inky liquid which, by the way, was used as a substitute for ink before artificial ink was invented, the reason and root of 'inky cap' name.

So, you can easily imagine how decomposing of shaggy mane mushrooms can stain everything in your world, including your hands. The process of darkening of shaggy mane mushrooms is called deliquescing. If you touch a mature shaggy mane mushroom, your hand will be stained with the distinctive inky-black color.

Fresh shaggy manes have a subtle earthy flavor and are excellent for pairing with chicken or in pasta. They are not great in strong-flavored dishes because their subtle taste will simply get lost.

As shaggy manes transform into the inky liquid, something magical happens. The flavor becomes more intense and aromatic than before. Some chefs use this gooey mass of deliquesced shaggy manes to make pasta dough though the process is quite tricky and may not be a good idea for novices to try.

Shaggy Mane Mushrooms Cooked with Parmesan (A Delicious Starter)

Ingredients:

- Shaggy mane mushrooms

- Eggs - beaten with some milk

- All-purpose flour

- Grated parmesan

- Fresh parsley (chopped)

- Salt and pepper - to taste

- Oil for frying

Directions:

Season the beaten egg with salt and pepper and add the chopped parsley to it. Use one hand for the wet coating and one for the dry coating. First, dip the shaggy mane mushrooms in the flour, then in the egg, and finally in the grated parmesan.

Heat the oil in a large skillet or non-stick surface until it is hot. Add the coated shaggy mane mushrooms to the hot oil and cook for about 2-3 minutes. The cheese might come off until the whole thing caramelizes into a cohesive mass of fried goodness.

Turn over the mushrooms and cook the other side for about 4-5 minutes or until they are cooked well. Remove from the oil, drain the excess in tissue paper, and serve immediately with a squeeze of lime juice.

Chapter Seven

Giant Puffballs and Boletes

Giant Puffballs

The giant puffball grows abundantly in places with a temperate climate. It grows in deciduous forests, fields, and meadows. Their harvest season is from later summer to early fall. Identifying characteristics of giant puffballs include:

- These mushrooms typically have a diameter ranging between 10 to 50 cm. Some are known to grow up to 150 cm too.

- A mature giant puffball has greenish-brown flesh. However, they are edible only at their early stage when the flesh is white. Mature giant puffballs must not be consumed. All species of giant puffballs can be eaten when young and are toxic when mature.

- The best way to make sure they can be eaten is to cut them open and check if the flesh is white.

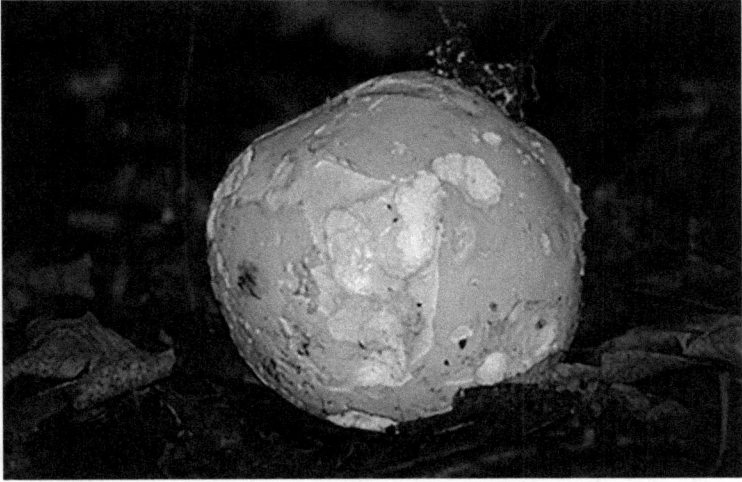

There are many toxic look-alikes of the young giant puffballs. A good way to ensure you have not picked the wrong one is to cut open the flesh. Edible puffballs have solid white interiors, whereas the toxic look-alikes have other colored interiors. Some toxic look-alikes might have white interiors. In such cases, you must also look for the silhouettes of gills or caps, and if you see them, then it is not an edible giant puffball.

Giant puffballs must not be washed because they soak up the water rapidly. They can be refrigerated for a few days without any loss to its edibility. There are multiple species of puffballs though the giant puffballs are the most common, kitchen-friendly, and obvious one. Some tips for harvesting giant puffballs:

- First, regardless of the size of the giant puffball, turn it over to make sure it is attached to the ground.

- Cut away the flesh from where it is attached to the ground and then inspect the mushroom.

- It is imperative that the puffball you have harvested is perfectly white. Yellowish or greenish spots means it is old and should not be consumed.

- If you notice a lot of tunneling on the puffball, then it could mean worms and insects.

- Cut through the flesh to see if the tunneling can be removed completely.

- Make sure all the bugs are removed to prevent them from continuing to eat your harvested puffball. If the remaining is firm and totally white, then you can take it home.

Cleaning giant puffballs are not very difficult, considering they have a leathery coating that protects them from grit and dirt. It is good to keep the skin on until the time of cooking them, especially if you plan to use the fresh specimens. The skin comes off quite easily. You can use your fingers or a paring knife to peel them off.

Puffballs turn rancid and emit an obnoxious smell like spoiled meat if left unattended a couple of days after picking up. It is, therefore, very important that you preserve them by chilling them. Of course, considering the size of giant puffballs, it makes sense to cut them into small chunks so that they fit into the refrigerator and chill them. Also, you can dry giant puffballs or turn them into a puree or hummus for later use.

Another creative way of preserving giant puffballs is to dry them, powder the dried mushrooms, and then use the powder to make unleavened bread. The pure white flesh of giant puffballs has the texture of marshmallows and the flavor of scallops. There are many ways you can cook giant puffballs. You can put them in soups and fry them in the batter. Or simply slice them and sauté them in a bit of butter. They are excellent substitutes for tofu. Grilling, frying, or broiling giant puffballs enhance the scallop-resembling flavor.

Classic Fried Giant Puffballs

Ingredients:

- Fresh giant puffball mushroom - 1 (thoroughly inspected and cleaned)
- Salt and pepper - to taste
- Cooking oil - for deep frying
- Breadcrumbs
- All-purpose flour
- Eggs - beaten with water or milk
- Any herbs of your choice
- Fresh lime juice

Directions:

Preheat your oven to 225-degrees-F. Season the flour with salt and pepper and cut the giant puffballs into ½-inch slices. Coat the slices with flour, beaten eggs, and breadcrumbs.

Heat the oil for deep frying. When it is sizzling hot, fry the puffballs slices until they are golden brown on both sides. Keep fried giant puffballs in the warmed oven until you finish frying all the slices. Then remove from the oven and serve with a sprinkling of your favorite herbs and a squeeze of lime.

Boletes

Boletes have pores and have a symbiotic relationship with their host. No species of boletes in North American are deadly or toxic. But, it is important not to give in to the false sense of security this information renders to beginners because although the inedible ones don't kill, their side-effects can be extremely unpleasant and grueling.

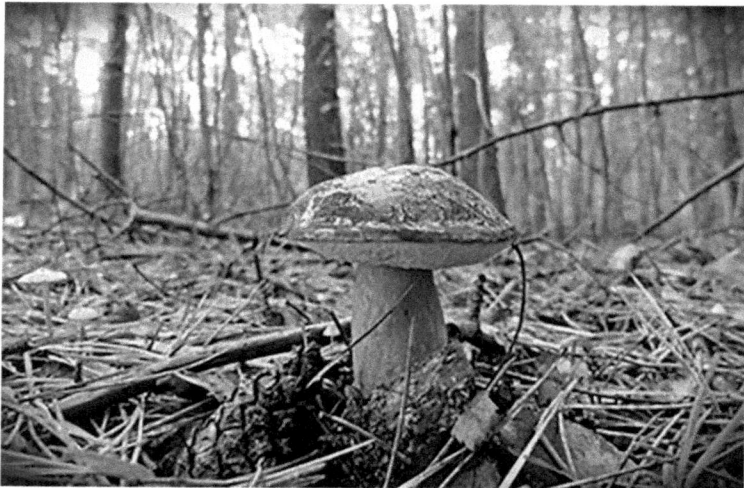

As a beginner, you must treat every species of mushrooms with care. In the initial stages, it is best not to consume any of your pickings until you have taken a second opinion from a trusted expert. Boletes are also known as porcini mushrooms and have multiple species. Here are identifying characteristics of boletes:

- They do not have gills, and the flesh is quite dense.

- The underside of the caps have pores from which the spores of boletes are scattered. The underside of the caps of boletes looks almost like a sponge.

- Boletes are known to be partial towards oak trees. You are likely to find them around oak trees more than any other kind of tree.

- The mycelium of boletes sprouts mushrooms during the rainy season and when the weather is cool. However, boletes do not thrive in winter months.

- The best season for harvesting boletes is during early fall.

Some tips to ensure you don't pick wrong inedible boletes:

When you pick a suspected bolete, crush or cut a corner of it. If it stains blue, then throw it away, especially if you are a beginner.

Some experts can tell the difference between edible and inedible blue-staining boletes too. For example, there is a two-color bolete species that stains blue and is edible too. However, as a beginner mushroom, any bolete that stains blue must not be consumed. Wait until you have reached that level of knowledge in mushroom foraging before consuming a blue-staining bolete.

If the bolete you picked up has yellow or bright red pores, then too, you must discard it. Many of the inedible varieties of boletes have pores under the caps that are yellow or brilliant red.

Bolete Julienne

Ingredients:

- Bolete mushrooms (cut into slices of ¼-inch thickness) - 4 ounces

- Cooking oil - 2 tbsp

- Onion (diced) - ¼ cup

- Garlic (diced) - 1 tbsp

- Unsalted butter - 1 tbsp

- All-purpose flour - 2 tbsp

- Sour cream - ½ cup

- Parmesan cheese - ¼ cup

- Grated gruyere - ¼ cup

Directions:

Preheat the oven to 375-degrees-F. Heat 1 tbsp oil until it is almost smoking. Add the boletes and cook over medium heat for 5 minutes until it is caramelized and browned, stirring occasionally. Remove the mushrooms from the heat and season with pepper and salt.

Now, add the remaining oil and fry the onions and garlic on low flame until tender. Add the cooked and seasoned boletes along with the juices formed while they were cooling in a bowl. Add the butter and wait for it to melt. Add the all-purpose flour and cook until the raw flavor of the flour is removed.

Add some wine to deglaze the pan and stir in the cheeses and the sour cream. The mixture would be creamy at this stage. Transfer it to a baking dish and bake until browned and bubbly. Typically, it would take about 15 minutes to bake this julienne.

Cool the baked dish for about 5-10 minutes before serving hot.

Chapter Eight

Ram's Head Mushrooms
and Bear's Head Tooth Mushrooms

Ram's Head Mushrooms

Ram's Head Mushrooms (Grifola frondosa) have different names, including **Hen of the Wood, Sheep's Head, Maitake**, and **Signoria**. You can find this variety of mushrooms at the base of many trees, especially oak trees in the northeastern parts of North America.

Foragers have reported finding this variety of mushroom as far as Idaho towards western North America. Ram's Head Mushrooms are also found in Japan and China. It is commonly used in Japanese cuisine. Maitake is the Japanese name, which means "the dancing mushroom."

Their harvest season is late summer to early fall after the rains. You need a large knife to harvest Ram's Head Mushrooms. It is best to harvest these mushrooms when they are young for optimal taste and texture. Hen of the Wood is parasitic mushrooms that live off-host trees, especially red and white oaks. You will see the Hen of the Wood form clusters that resemble cauliflower florets.

Although Ram's Head Mushrooms have a short lifespan, they are perennial mushrooms that keep growing in the same place repeatedly year after year. Identifying characteristics include:

- This mushroom grows as a large coral-like clump. It grows in circular layers from a common branch of a living tree. It's tongue-like fronds form a cauliflower shape, and you get to see rosettes of this mushroom under hardwood trees, especially oak trees.

- The caps are grayish-brown that are either curled or have the shape of a spoon.

- In Japan, some varieties of this mushroom can grow up to 100 pounds!

- The stems are white in color and have branches.

- As the mushrooms, they become quite tough

Ram's Head Mushrooms taste great when sautéed in olive oil or butter. Here are some tips for scouring for hen of the wood mushrooms:

- You can find them in your local park if there are old oak trees. Considering that it is a park, you must be ready to be disappointed that someone faster than you have already picked them.

- You can use a bike to forage for this mushroom instead of hiking because you can cover a lot more ground at a faster rate, thereby helping you collect easily discoverable hens-of-the-woods quickly. Using a bike will also help you be ahead of other foragers who tend to hike rather than use a bike.

- If you find one, then you just need to look in the neighborhood, and you are likely to find a lot more. Look at the base of oak trees, and once you have found a cluster under one tree, you can keep returning to the same place and rest assured you will find hens year on year unfailingly. Interestingly, they keep returning to the same tree every year during the fruiting season.

- Also, if you find one tree, then the neighboring trees are also likely to be infected. Remember, they are parasitic mushrooms.

When you find a young hen-of -the-wood which is usually the size of a golf ball, the tendency is to wait for it to become bigger, considering they can grow to very large sizes. But, it is important to know that young and tender against old and tough are better to pick.

Bigger is not necessarily better when it comes to ram's head mushroom. When you see a hen-of-the-wood, then just take it without giving in to the natural urge of waiting for a week to 'hopefully get a bonanza." The chances of your mushroom getting infected by larvae, slugs, and beetles are high. Not only this, but the cleanliness of the mushroom is compromised too because as it grows, this mushroom tends to absorb physical dirt into its flesh, especially during rains.

Cleaning such dirty mushrooms can be quite tricky. In fact, people have found pebbles and insects lodged deep inside the flesh of some large-sized maitake. You must thoroughly inspect and examine every maitake you pick before you cook them. One good thing about maitakes is that they are generally free of worms. Just inspect them to ensure they are totally germ-free.

Large-sized ram's head mushrooms are the best cut into bite-sized pieces before cleaning and cooking them. Inspect the bite-sized pieces for grit, grime, and sometimes, even insects. The younger, smaller ones can be cleaned and cooked as a whole without cutting them. Roasting these small-sized maitakes is like roasting a piece of meat.

Pickling and sautéing with freezing are great preservation methods for ram's head mushrooms. The dried ones can be powdered and used to make mushroom stock whenever needed.

Fried Ram's Head Mushrooms

Ingredients:

- Ram's head mushrooms

- Milk - ⅓ to ½ cup

- All-purpose flour - ½ cup

- Seasoned bread crumbs - ½ cup

- Oil for deep frying

Directions:

Combine milk, eggs, flour, and breadcrumbs. Use more milk if needed to make sure the batter is of the right consistency, neither too thick nor too thin.

Heat oil in a skillet. Fry the mushrooms coated with the batter in medium heat until golden brown.

Serve hot.

Bear's Head Tooth Mushrooms

Bear's Head Tooth Mushrooms (Hericium americanum) is also referred to as **Pom-Pom mushrooms, Monkey's Head, Lion's Mane**, and **Bearded Hedgehog** mushroom. They are commonly found all over the world, especially in deciduous and alpine forests. It has a shaggy appearance and is native to the eastern parts of North America, especially in the east of the Rocky Mountains.

There are four species found in North America, all of which are edible. There are no poisonous look-alikes identified in North America yet. They grow very well on rotten logs as well in injured parts of living hardwood trees in shaded areas. The harvest season is autumn. Identifying characteristics:

- This mushroom looks as if numerous icicles are hanging or dangling from the log or the strong, sturdy stalks of the mushroom. This distinctive feature makes this mushroom stand apart.

- The tooth-like appendages of this mushroom grow on tree branches and form a mop-like structure with the appearance of dangling spines.

- This mushroom is white in color, though, as it matures, the teeth take on a brownish or yellowish tinge.

- The spores are white in color.

All the white parts of Bear's Head Tooth Mushroom are edible. They should be eaten only in the immature stage. They taste great when cooked in butter and can also be used in soups. The taste of the bear's head tooth mushroom is comparable to that of lobsters. This mushroom pairs very well with corn, potatoes, cabbage, garlic, shallots, leeks, onions, and meats like beef, pork, and chicken.

The thing to remember is that once picked; these mushrooms have to be consumed within a day or two. They become bitter even if stored in the refrigerator. Bear's head tooth mushrooms are rich in Vitamin D, iron, fiber, protein, and antioxidants. The Indian tribes of North America used dried and powdered bear's head tooth mushrooms to heal wounds and cuts.

Mixed Wild Mushrooms with Parsley and Garlic

Ingredients:

- Mixed wild mushrooms - 8 ounces

- Salt and pepper - to taste

- Fresh garlic (chopped) - ½ tsp

- Cooking oil - 2 tbsp

- Fresh parsley (chopped) - 1 tsp

- Unsalted butter - 1 tsp

Directions:

Heat the oil in a large pan until it is hot. Now, reduce the flame to medium heat, add the mushrooms and cook with salt and pepper until the mushrooms are caramelized. Next, add garlic, butter, and parsley. Cook for one more minute, stirring continuously to make sure the seasonings are distributed evenly. Remove from oil and serve hot.

Chapter Nine

Reishi Mushrooms
and Chicken of the Wood

Reishi Mushrooms

Reishi mushrooms are one of the best and easiest mushrooms for a beginner forager to start his or her foraging journey. They are easy to identify and do not have any toxic look-alikes making them relatively safe for picking and consumption. Reishi mushrooms are a bit tough to eat. But, their medicinal values are excellently backed by plenty of scientific research. Reishi mushrooms are also known by other names including:

- Lingzhi

- Mushroom of immortality

- Herb of spiritual potency

- 10000-year mushroom

- Artists' conk

- Varnish self

Many varieties of Reishi mushrooms exist all around the globe, although their medicinal benefits and properties are more or less the same, regardless of their geography. All the species grow on dead and dying trees. These fungi fruit annually (harvest season is in summer), and like many other species, once you find them on any dead and decaying stump of a dying tree, you can keep coming back to that location each year during the harvest season and find new fruiting bodies growing there. This will continue until all the nutrients from the stump are used up by the mycelium.

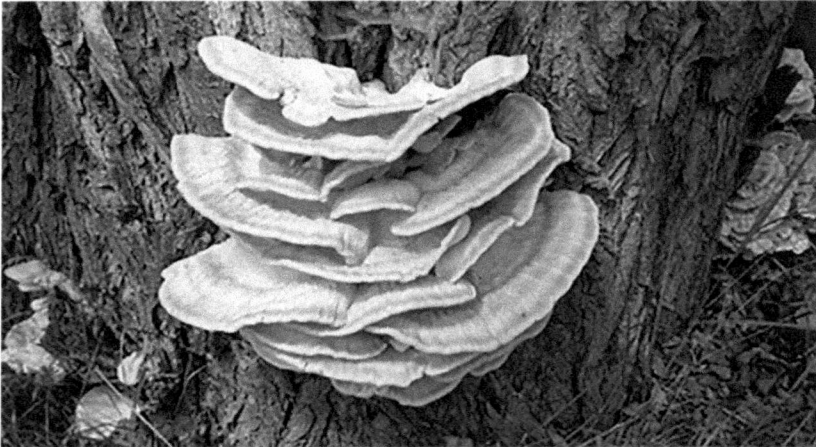

Identifying characteristics of Reishi mushrooms are:

- They are a fan- or kidney-shaped and have a distinctive color ranging between red and orange.

- The top of the mushroom has a lacquered, shiny finish.

- There are no gills, and the underside of the cap is white when young, which gets gray or tan as the mushrooms mature. The underside of the cap also has tiny pink dots resembling pinpricks.

- Reishi mushrooms grow horizontally out of the wood stump or log.

- The stems are either very short or completely absent.

- Reishi mushrooms have a strong woody, though pleasant smell. Some people think the smell is similar to decomposing leaf mulch.

- Spores come out from the underside of the caps. The spore print of Reishi mushrooms is brown. You can also find spores on the logs as well as the caps of the lower mushrooms as the spores from the upper ones fall on them. The sprinkling of spores from the upper mushrooms tends to dull the red-orange color of the caps.

- The flesh of the mushroom becomes tan or brown when bruised. The characteristic red-orange cap of hemlock Reishi variety is visible as it matures.

- Commonly, Reishi mushrooms are 4 to 6 inches in width and about 0.5 to 1 inch in thickness. However, some of them can grow to about 2 inches in thickness and up to a foot in width.

- Most Reishi mushrooms do not last for more than a few days because as they mature, slugs begin to devour them.

It is important to harvest only those mushrooms whose cap's underside is white. Molds tend to grow on the tanned/browned and mature Reishi mushrooms. Also, as these mushrooms can bruise quite rapidly after harvesting, preserving them quickly is important too. You can easily identify the new and young white mushrooms as they emerge from the mycelium.

There are multiple species of Reishi mushrooms and the ones found in North America are:

Ganoderma lucidum - This species is a common ingredient in Chinese medicine and grows in warmer climates such as Asia, southern Europe, and the South Pacific. In North America, you can find this species of Reishi mushrooms in the Southeastern US.

Ganoderma curtisii - This species of Reishi mushrooms can be found from Massachusetts up to Nebraska. With a distinctive ochre-colored cap, this species has a matte rather than a shiny lacquer finish on top. Mostly, it is found on maple and oak logs. But these mushrooms also grow on other hardwoods.

Ganoderma tsugae - This species is commonly referred to as hemlock Reishi or sometimes as hemlock varnish shelf. Tsugae means hemlock, which is an indicator of where these mushrooms commonly grow. Although hemlock trees are typical hosts for this species of Reishi mushrooms, you can also find them on birch or maple trees, especially those that are close to hemlock trees. You will find the freshest hemlock Reishi mushrooms between May and July.

As mentioned earlier, there are no toxic look-alikes of Reishi mushrooms, which makes them one of the ideal mushrooms for novice foragers. It can, however, be quite a difficult task to distinguish between the various species of Reishi mushrooms. However, all of them are cooked and preserved in the same way. Also, the nutritional benefits of all the species are the same. The subtle differences between the species are more for academics than mushroom consumers.

Just to reiterate a point mentioned earlier, pick only young Reishi mushrooms that have white undersides and bright caps. The older mushrooms with dull caps and brownish or tanned undersides tend to have a lot of potentially harmful molds and should not be eaten.

You can either pull the mushroom gently from the host tree or use a knife to cut the softer specimens. Also, you must make sure you are not picking mushrooms growing around other toxic plants, trees, and vegetation, especially poison ivy, which can sometimes be found close by.

A word of caution about consuming Reishi for people who are on other medications, especially for the liver. There are records of allergic reactions when Reishi and certain liver medications are combined. But, the reactions stopped immediately after Reishi was discontinued.

They have to be quickly dried because they spoil rapidly. Dried Reishi mushrooms should be stored in airtight containers away from direct sunlight. You can also make a mushroom tincture with Reishi mushrooms immediately after harvesting them. They have both alcohol-soluble and water-soluble constituents in them. Therefore, a double extraction method of tincture preparation will ensure you get optimal medicinal benefits of this wonderful species.

As a medicine, the best way to consume Reishi mushrooms is to make a strong tea with thinly sliced mushrooms simmered for about 1-2 hours in water. The dried mushrooms can be powdered and used in other dishes or put into Reishi capsules and taken daily to boost your immunity.

Reishi Mushroom Vegetable Soup

Ingredients:

- Olive oil - 1 tbsp

- Onion (diced) - 1

- Garlic cloves (minced) - 4

- Peeled and grated fresh ginger - 2 tbsp

- Carrots (sliced) - 2

- Fennel bulb (diced) - 1

- A mixture of wild mushrooms (sliced) - 4 cups

- Water - 6 cups

- Reishi mushroom powder - ¼ cup

- Miso paste - ¼ cup

- Allspice - 1 tbsp

- Fresh thyme - 1 tbsp

- Kale (chopped) - 3 cups

- Salt and pepper - to taste

Directions:

Heat oil in a large pot and add onions to the heated oil. Sauté for 2 minutes. Then add garlic and sauté for another minute. Then add the ginger and all the other chopped veggies. Reishi powder should not be added at this time. Sauté this mixture for 5 minutes.

Now, add the water, dry spices, miso paste, and Reishi powder. Bring the liquid mixture to a boil. Reduce the flame to a simmer and cook the broth for about an hour. Lastly, add the kale into the hot broth to wilt. Add the required salt and pepper, and your Reishi mushroom vegetable soup is ready.

Chicken of the Wood Mushrooms

Also known as chicken mushrooms, sulfur shelf mushrooms are found growing on adult trees as well as dead ones, especially on the eastern side of the Rocky Mountains. While the most typical harvest season is summer, they can also be harvested right from spring until summer, provided the climate is right for its growth. Identifying characteristics include:

- Sulfur shelf mushrooms do not have gills.

- The upper part of this mushroom is salmon-pink or orange in color, while the lower part is bright yellow.

- They grow in clumps on many trees, but especially on oak trees. It is important that you recognize the host tree before picking sulfur shelf mushrooms because they are toxic if they grow on some specific trees

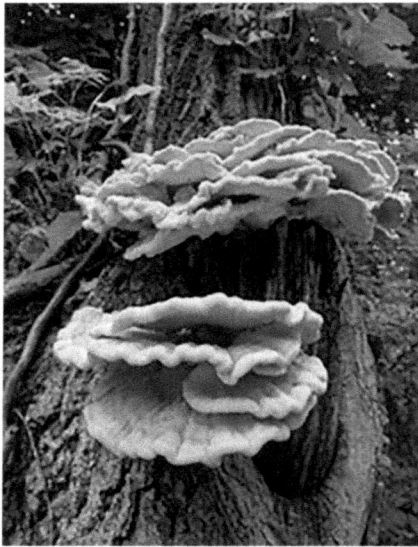

Sulfur shelf mushrooms growing on pine, spruce, juniper, eucalyptus, hemlock, fir, tamarack, or locust trees are poisonous look-alikes. The ones growing on oak trees are the safest. Therefore, if you cannot identify the host tree because it is dead, then it is safest for you not to pick the mushroom.

Moreover, only the young caps of sulfur shelf mushrooms can be cooked and eaten. The stem, as well as the more mature of these mushrooms, are too tough to be cooked. The caps of the young ones are popular for their rich and meaty flavor.

The vibrant yellow colors and the impressive size make it very easy to identify the chicken of the wood mushrooms. With a meaty, lemony flavor, the reason for its name is that this mushroom tastes similar to chicken. Some people tend to think that the taste of this mushroom is more aligned with lobster or crab.

Regardless of which meat it tastes similar to, there is no denying the fact that the chicken of the wood mushroom is a delectable substitute for meat, and mushroom eaters love it. Chicken mushrooms can take the place of tofu or chicken in any recipe. One important point of concern is that some people tend to have gastric issues when they consume this mushroom. So, try eating a small amount for the first time, and if you are fine with it, then you can go ahead and consume it without fear.

Also, it is important to remember NOT to pick chicken mushrooms growing on eucalyptus, cedar, or coniferous trees as these are known to contain toxins that could create problems for some people. Here are some basic facts about chicken of the wood mushrooms before we move into a more detailed understanding of identifying characteristics:

- There are many species of the chicken of the woods mushrooms. They can be saprophytic or parasitic fungi. You are most likely to find them at the base of a living or a dead tree.

- They have a distinctive yellowish-orange color that makes it very easy to identify them. They normally grow in large clusters of overlapping brackets. The yellowish-orange color fades as the mushrooms mature.

- Other names of chicken of the wood are sulfur shelf, chicken fungus, and chicken mushroom. They belong to the genus Laetiporus.

- There are currently about 12 different species of chicken mushrooms. Some of them include Laetiporus sulphureus, Laetiporus cincinnatus (both found on Eastern North America), Laetiporus gilbertsonii (found on the west coast of North America), and Laetiporus conifericola (found in Western North America).

Considered a 'safe' mushroom for beginners, chickens can be easily identified with the following characteristic features:

- This mushroom does not have a stem, and therefore, there is no height to talk about.

- The caps themselves grow into large-sized brackets ranging from 2 to 10 inches in diameter and up to 10 inches in length.

- The fan-shaped brackets can be smooth or slightly wrinkled. The brackets grow in an overlapping pattern and appear stacked on top of each other. Therefore, the entire fruiting body can become quite large.

- Both the outside as well as the inside of the cap are yellowish-orange in color. With age, the brightness of the flesh, as well as colors of the exterior, fades. Also, mature chicken mushrooms tend to have hard and crumbly flesh.

- There are no gills under the caps, only yellowish or whitish pores from which the spores are dispersed. As the caps are clustered together and not distinct, it is not easy to get spores of chicken mushrooms.

Chicken mushrooms always grow at or on the base of living or dead trees. They never grow out directly from the soil or the ground. Mostly, they grow on dying or dead hardwoods, especially oak, although you can find them at the base of beech and cherry trees as well. Chickens growing on cedar and eucalyptus should be avoided as they have the potential to cause gastric distress.

They can be harvested from summer right through fall, which means you will find a lot of chickens mushrooming between August and October. In warmer climates, you can find them even in early winter months too. Some general cooking tips for chicken mushrooms:

As these mushrooms become harder and brittle as they age, young specimens work best in your dishes. Look for tender and juicy caps that ooze a liquid when you cut them. Also, the margins of the brackets are better for cooking than the centers which have a woody or corky flavor, which is not necessarily pleasant to eat. Because they are so spongy and light, it is best to clean them with a damp cloth as regular washing might result in water-logging them.

They can be refrigerated in a paper bag for not more than a week. Cut them into small, bite-sized pieces before cooking them. You can blanch, fry, sauté, or bake them. You can preserve them by sautéing and freezing them for later use. Another important point to remember is to be careful with the amount of oil you use while cooking chickens. They tend to absorb a lot of oil, giving you stomach issues later on.

Pasta Sauce with Chicken of the Woods Mushrooms

Ingredients:

- Butter - 4 tbsps

- Young chicken mushrooms (cleaned and chopped finely) - 1 pound

- Shallots (finely chopped) - 1

- Sherry or dry white wine - ¼ cup

- Milk - 1 cup

- Vegetable stock - 1 cup

- Flour - 3 tbsp

- Dried or fresh sprigs of thyme

- Salt and pepper

Directions:

Melt the butter in a pan and cook the shallots and mushrooms, stirring continuously. First, the mushroom will release their liquids, and then they will reabsorb it. This process will take about 10 minutes.

Next, add the wine and cook for another 5-10 minutes. Mix the stock and milk and bring to a boil, and then simmer slowly.

In another pot, melt the remaining butter. Stir in the flour slowly and cook for about 4 minutes. Remove from the heat and whisk in the simmering stock/milk mixture, taking a little amount at a time. Adding the entire liquid will create a big messy clump.

Add the thyme to this sauce and put it back on the stove to cook for another 4-5 minutes, all the while stirring vigorously to prevent lumping. Now, mix in the mushrooms and season with salt and pepper. This sauce can be served with any pasta of your choice. You may not need too much cheese in your pasta dish if you use this sauce.

Chapter Ten

Black Trumpet Mushrooms and Chaga Mushrooms

Black Trumpet Mushrooms

You can find black trumpet mushrooms all across North America, mostly in mossy hardwood forests where oak and beech grow abundantly. Other names of this mushroom are **"horn of plenty,"** **"devil's horn," "devil's trumpet**, and **"trumpet of death."** Another name is **"black chanterelles"** because they are closely related to chanterelles.

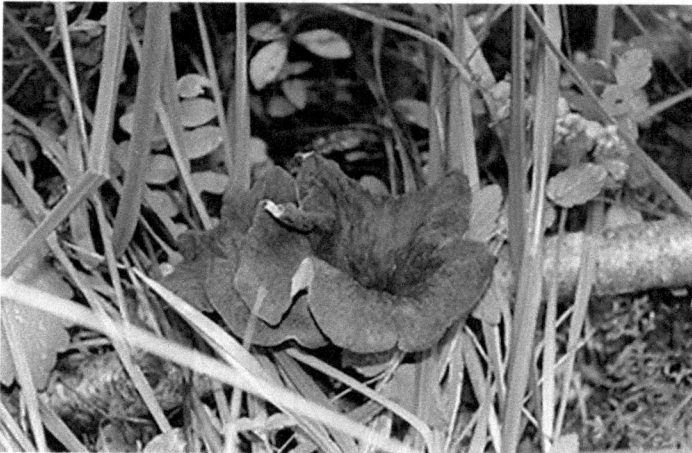

Most often, these mushrooms are found near streams and washes as they prefer damp and dark spaces. Their harvest season is in summer and fall, although they are found even in winters in the southern parts of North America. You are likely to find black trumpet mushrooms in Californian foraging areas, even in winters. Identifying characteristics include:

- Black trumpet mushrooms grow in leaf litter, which is why they are quite hard to find.

- They mostly grow in clusters, although there are rare cases of one mushroom growing alone.

- The cap of the black trumpet mushroom can be gray, dark-brown, or inky black. The caps are shaped like a trumpet or vase, which is the reason they are named so.

- The underside of the cap is smooth and has no gills, teeth, or pores. The top part of the cap might have scales but mostly has a smooth although slightly wrinkled feel.

The best part of this mushroom is that it does not have a toxic look-alike, which makes it a perfect mushroom for novice foragers to find and pick. The black trumpet mushrooms have a smoky and rich flavor. They have to be wiped clean thoroughly because they get quite dirty.

You can give them a quick rinse, but you must avoid drowning them. Black trumpet mushrooms hold their flavor very well even when they are dried. They taste delicious when sautéed with oil and garlic. They can be powdered and sprinkled on cooked grains and soups to enhance the flavor of the dishes.

Black trumpet mushrooms with their rich, smoky flavor and fruity, pleasant aroma are gourmet edibles. While they are a great mushroom species for beginner foragers considering there are no poisonous look-alikes, it is not easy to find them because of their dark color and irregular shape.

To a novice eye, the dark and irregular appearance of black trumpet mushrooms makes the forest floor look like it has multiple little holes. Many beginners have missed these gourmet ingredients completely despite seeing them right in front of their eyes. So, they are easy to identify but difficult to find. Some basic facts about black trumpet mushrooms:

- The most common species of black trumpet mushrooms is Craterellus cornucopioides, and another not-so-common species is Craterellus foetidus.

- They are funnel- or vase-shaped and are of black, brown, or gray color. The cap edges are rolled inwards and have a wavy, trumpet-like appearance.

- They have no gills or any other spore-bearing structure, including teeth or pores. The underside of the caps is either smooth or slightly wrinkled. You are likely to get a soft feel when you touch them, comparable to touching suede.

- The stem of black trumpet mushrooms grow to a few inches in height and are usually the same color as the cap, or maybe, slightly lighter.

- The stem is hollow on the inside, can break easily, and the flesh is quite thin. Experts are still not sure about the category of fungi they belong to. They are considered to be both saprophytic as well as symbiotic fungi.

Considering the difficulty in locating black trumpet mushrooms because they camouflage so well into the forest floor, use these tips to make sure you don't miss a treasure for want of not paying attention to the "holes on the forest floor."

- Hardwood forests, especially oak and beech trees, are the most common places black trumpets grow in. These mushrooms do not grow on the wood directly but close to it. You are not likely to find black trumpet mushrooms at the base of trees, but again, close to it.

- They are likely to fruit in green mossy areas. The green color of the moss makes it easy to locate these dark-colored mushrooms.

- Black trumpet mushrooms are attracted to damp and dark places, and therefore, look hard near small streams and washes, especially on the edge of streams flowing through hills.

- As you walk on your mushroom foraging trail, remember to walk slowly and look directly down. It is very easy to miss them unless you are standing over and crushing them with your shoe-laden feet. Look minutely, closely, and slowly, especially when you are examining leaf litter.

Black trumpet mushrooms grow in clusters. Therefore, if you have managed to locate one, then look even more closely in the nearby areas, and you are likely to find many more. Also, as there are no toxic look-alikes, they are relatively safe for beginner foragers. However, it is a wise decision to take a second opinion before eating them, regardless of how safe the mushroom species is believed to be.

This species of mushrooms have an excellent rich and smoky flavor and are a great addition in many recipes. You can add them to pasta, soups, seafood dishes, and more and experience the flavor of your dish taken to gourmet levels.

Drying black trumpet mushrooms are a great way to preserve them, considering they hold their rich flavor when dried. Dried mushrooms can be powered or chopped and added to your dishes. They are great to flavor rice, couscous, butter, and even white wines.

It is wise to clean foraged black trumpet mushrooms before cooking them. Tear them apart gently, and wipe the insides and the outsides clean. A quick rinse is okay if they are very gritty. The thinness of the flesh is an excellent deterrent for bugs and insects, and therefore, you will rarely find these mushrooms infected. However, snails and slugs enjoy this mushroom. Sometimes, you might find some insects and spiders make their home within the funneled cap of these mushrooms. Make sure your mushroom is totally clean before cooking them.

The closest look-alike of black trumpet mushrooms is the blue chanterelles. Blue chanterelles are also edible and share the vase-shaped cap as well as the absence of gills with black trumpets. Pig's ears mushrooms (also edible) resemble black trumpets too. The devil's urn (another edible though not recommended for beginners because of their toughness) can also be confused with black trumpets.

Monkfish with Black Trumpet Sauce and Spinach

Ingredients:

- Monkfish - 1 pound

- Fresh black trumpet mushrooms - ¼ pound

- Fresh spinach - 1 pound

- Butter - 3 tbsp

- Shallot - 1 (minced)

- Scotch - ¼ cup

- Heavy cream - ½ cup

- Olive oil - 2 tbsp

- Salt and pepper - to taste

Directions:

Clean the monkfish and cut into ½-inch fillets. Rinse and clean black trumpet mushrooms, drain and squeeze them dry. Cut large-sized mushrooms into bite-sized pieces.

Melt butter in a pan, sauté the shallots for a minute, then add the cleaned and cut mushrooms. Add the scotch and cook until the mushrooms become tender. Then add the cream and cook until the mushrooms are all coated well with the cream. Season with salt and pepper and keep aside.

Next, cook the spinach until the leaves wilt. Remove from heat, drain and squeeze out all the extra water, and keep aside.

In another pan, cook the monkfish on high almost-smoking heat with some salt and pepper. You would need about 4-5 minutes to cook each side of the fish. Lay the cooked monkfish on a plate filled with the cooked spinach. Then, pour the mushroom sauce over the fish-n-spinach and serve.

Chaga Mushrooms

For centuries now, Chaga mushrooms have been foraged from the wild and used as a medicinal remedy for multiple illnesses ranging from high blood pressure to cancer. Despite the abundant availability of these mushrooms all over the world, Chaga mushrooms are quite pricey.

Chaga mushrooms are commonly found on white and yellow birches, and when you find one birch with these mushrooms, you are likely to find more in the vicinity. They grow abundantly in the world in northern climates, such as in North America, northern Europe, China, and Russia. They are best and easiest to harvest in winters where the trees are free of dense foliage that can obstruct your view. These black-colored mushrooms tend to stand out in the white snow as well as against the light-colored barks of birch trees.

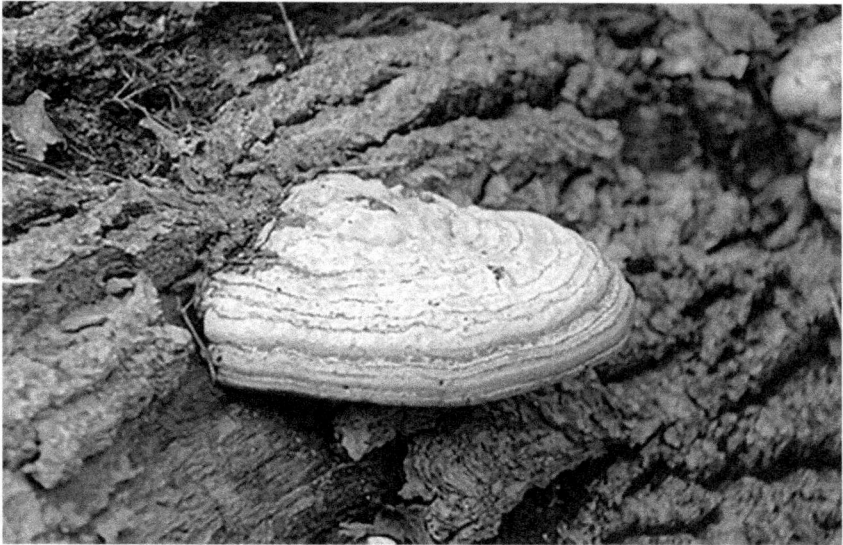

Chaga is replete with multiple nutrients, including antioxidants, minerals, and phytonutrients, which is the reason they are regularly used as therapeutics in different cultures around the world. Chaga mushrooms have a high content of betulinic acid, the reason why they are believed to be useful to treat or reduce the symptoms of even some forms of cancers. However, there is not enough scientific evidence to back such claims thought studies continue to be carried out. The relevance of the miracle cure is not an important one for mushroom foragers. Chaga mushrooms are excellently nutritious and liked by mushroom lovers.

Although winters are the best time to forage for Chaga mushrooms, they can be found all year round in North America. It is a parasitic mushroom that feeds on the wood of yellow and white birch trees. Once the mycelium gets hold of the nutrition from these trees, mushrooms start to grow and come out from the tree barks in the form of a black (because it is loaded with melanin) conk or tumor.

To prevent harvesting the wrong mushroom species, it is safest to identify and harvest Chaga mushrooms only from living birch trees. Chaga mushrooms and the host birch trees live together for about 30 years by which time, the tree's nutrients are completely depleted, and it dies. When the tree dies, so does the Chaga mushrooms that grew on them. Therefore, you must not pick Chaga mushrooms from dead trees.

You can use a knife, hatchet, or ax to break off a chunk of Chaga mushrooms or the entire bark on which they are growing. You must leave a bit of the bark in place so that new Chaga mushrooms can grow from there. Harvested Chaga can be consumed in the form of tea or preserved as a tincture for later use. Use these steps to clean, dry, and make Chaga mushroom tea or tincture/extract:

- Rinse the harvested mushrooms in water to remove all debris, grit, and insects or slugs that could be hiding in the small, unreachable crevices.

- Then, cut or break the Chaga mushrooms into smaller bits for faster drying as well as to prevent molding.

- Next, dry these small pieces in a cool and dry place until they are bone dry, a process that could take up to a month.

- You can cut up the dried mushrooms into smaller pieces or grind them into a fine powder. You can store the pieces and the powder for a long time as long as you ensure that they are totally dry and are kept in airtight containers.

You can add the pieces or powder to your dishes or make tea. The larger pieces are great for making tea rather than for flavoring your stews and other dishes. And the best part is that you can reuse these large pieces of dried Chaga mushrooms to repeatedly make tea until you don't get a rich dark liquid with them.

Simple Chaga Tea Recipe for Beginners

Ingredients:
- Ground or powdered Chaga - 1 tsp

- Maple syrup or honey - to taste

- Lemon

Directions:
Chaga tea is the best way to get all the medicinal benefits of this wonder mushroom. Put one teaspoon of Chaga powder (you can add one tbsp if you want it stronger) into a teacup. Add hot water into the

cup and keep it covered for about 5-10 minutes, which is the best way for the Chaga to be infused into the water. Filter out the Chaga tea. Then you can add maple syrup or honey along with a dash of lime. Stir it well, and your tea is ready.

Chapter Eleven

Best Places in North America for Mushroom Foraging

The first few generations of people to exist on Earth only wanted to survive. They would consume anything, be it animal or vegetable, in order to satisfy their hunger. In the twenty-first century, people have become very finicky about where they get their food from. We want to know exactly what is going in our food and where it is coming from. The only way we can be sure of such things is if we grow and forage our own food.

If this is your first time foraging, it is best to do lots of research or, better yet, consult an expert. You might stumble upon a beautiful cluster of mushrooms that are actually poisonous. So it is important to know exactly what you want before going on your mushroom hunt.

Mushroom hunting can develop into a hobby very quickly. All it takes is some patience and a few inexpensive tools. Chefs pay good money for well-harvested mushrooms, including some delicious species like chanterelles, morels, and porcinis.

There are certain conditions which places must satisfy before becoming suitable for mushroom growth.

- **Proper climate**: it is vital for the region you want to grow your mushrooms to have a suitable climate. The region must be located in either of the temperate zones with ambient humidity and rainfall.

- **Proximity to wooden areas:** mushrooms play a very important role in keeping forests alive. If not for mushrooms, the dead matter would never decay, and soon the forest would be covered with debris of dead matter. Keeping this in mind, parks and rainforests are places where mushroom growth is certain.

Although many of the North American states are rich in mushrooms, people can't casually walk into forests and pick out the mushrooms they like. If someone owns the land they want to forage, they have written consent from the land's owner. And yet, people are allowed to pick up only some species of mushrooms. Other mushroom species are rare and are meant to be preserved.

Mushrooms are mostly meant only for personal use. But the government does allow some mushrooms to be sold in the market, including Hedgehog, Porcini, Pacific Golden Chanterelle, Oyster, Saffron Milk Cap, etc.

In the case of mushroom poisoning, it is recommended to keep a sample of the mushroom which the patient consumed so that finding an antidote would be quick, and treatment would be done before it is too late.

Here are a few places in North America where you are guaranteed to forage and feast on mushrooms.

Weyerhaeuser, Wisconsin

If you plan on visiting Wisconsin for your mushroom hunt, meet Samuel Thayer. This wild food expert takes and leads foraging classes from May to October with events and discussions during Winter.

During spring, morels are found in abundance in Wisconsin. During the first few days of Spring, morel mushrooms are typically found in the slopes which point to the sun. They grow near dead Ash, apple, or elm trees. In summer, you will come across a lot of chanterelles.

Porcini or king boletes are also found in abundance in Wisconsin in the summer months. These large mushrooms that can grow over a foot in width and weigh more than a pound, porcinis are usually found under oak and spruce trees from late June up to September right across the state of Wisconsin.

New York City, New York

When you are in New York City and want to go mushroom hunting, make sure to consult Steve Brill in Central Park before doing so. You can spend the day with him discovering different and edible species of mushrooms in the city that never sleeps. These tours happen during most March to December, and depending on the season during which you go for the tour, you will get to see different species of mushrooms.

When people go mushroom hunting in New York City, they will come across a large variety of mushroom species. They taste best when they are eaten with butter and garlic. During summer, chanterelles are something you would see every day. It is important to be able to differentiate between the poisonous Jack o' Lantern and chanterelle mushrooms. They look very similar on the outside, and the transition is clear only if you cut one of them lengthwise and notice how their gills are arranged.

Also, the New York Mycological Society organizes foraging expeditions almost every weekend. The foragers gather together looking for both edible and poisonous versions. The edible ones are used for cooking up some delicious meals, and the toxic ones are used to enhance the knowledge and skill of members so that they can teach novices what mushrooms to keep off their dinner plate.

Ithaca, New York

Elevate your camping standards to glamorous and colorful firelit and safari-themed tours. You will have nothing to worry about if you go camping with Sarah Kelsen in Buttermilk Falls State Park in Ithaca, New York.

All it takes is ninety minutes for you to be fully capable of differentiating between a large variety of plants and mushrooms. Sarah encourages her tour group to taste the medicinal properties of the mushrooms and plants, which you will find during the tour. She is also open to questions. Sarah conducts her tours between April and November.

The Cornell Mushroom Club of the Cornell University College of Agriculture and Life Sciences allows membership to people living in and around Ithaca, New York. The members get to know about mushroom foraging events and regular information-filled newsletters. Here are some details of what kind of mushrooms you can forage for in respective seasons in Ithaca:

- State forests, wildlife areas, forest preserves, and other multiple-use vegetation areas - allowed for recreational mushroom foraging for personal use. Banned for commercial foraging.

- State parks - are out of bounds for all kinds of mushroom foraging.

Morels are found in plenty in May. King boletes can be found in June under white spruce trees. Chanterelles are commonly seen in July if you look closely at the base of oak trees. In August and September, you will find a lot of giant puffballs. From September and right through winter, you will find many varieties of mushrooms in Ithaca, New York.

McCloud, California

California is the #1 destination for mushroom hunters. In fact, McCloud has an entire music festival dedicated to the mushroom called McCloud Mushroom and Music Festival. Todd Spanier knew locally as the "King of Mushrooms" leads an enthusiastic team on an exciting mushroom hunt during the festival, an event highlight that many novice and experienced foragers don't like to miss. There are multiple workshops teaching all things connected to mushroom foraging. While here, the multi-course mushroom dinner is a must-attend event too, which consists of tasting gourmet mushroom dishes.

Chesterfield, Missouri

Chesterfield is located very close to the Mark Twain National Forest, where different mushroom species are found in abundance. They have an entire season dedicated to morel mushrooms called 'Morel Madness.'

The time you pick to go mushrooms, hunting will affect the mushrooms you come back home with. If you go during Spring, you will find a lot of morels, and if you go during Summer, you will end up finding a lot of chanterelles. But whichever mushrooms you come back with, there is no way you will not enjoy them if you sauté butter and thyme and have them over a grilled steak.

Eugene, Oregon

The city of Eugene is surrounded by old, giant forests with conifers, ferns, and fungi. The Willamette, Mt. Hood, and Siuslaw National Forests are within short driving distances from Eugene. You can always approach the Cascade Mythological Society if you want help with your first mushroom hunt.

There is a strict rule in Oregon where mushrooms can be harvested for personal use only. Eugene is filled with lush, green forests with moderate temperature and rainfall; perfect for mushroom growth.

The Tillamook State Forest and Siuslaw National Forest cover large areas of land, which are prime territories for mushrooms.

Hot Springs, North Carolina

The Hot Springs is located very close to the Appalachian Trail, which has a high potential for successful mushroom hunts. If you drive just forty-five minutes southeast to Asheville, you can attend the monthly meetings of the Asheville Mushroom Club, where you can connect with other excited mushroom hunters and exchange ideas.

The entire Appalachian Trail is covered with thick temperate, woody rainforests. The range stretches from northeastern Alabama all the way up to New Brunswick. This area is not home only to a large species of mushrooms but is also known for other wild delicacies such as ramps, fiddlehead ferns, and wild berries during spring.

Mendocino, California

Mendocino is just a three-hour drive north from the Bay area on California's coast. The Mendocino Coast Botanical Gardens hosts a mushroom walk every Monday during November and December, and they host a weeklong event known as Mushroom Feast Mendocino.

Once you start going deep into the forests of California, you will find small patches of mushrooms. Golden chanterelles take up most of the territory. You might come across candy cap mushrooms too, which are often used in baked goods. They taste very similar to maple syrup.

Olympia, Washington

The pacific northwest is a must-visit for both beginner and professional mushroom hunters of the world. Olympia is conveniently located next to forests with decomposing natural materials. Also, around the area, you will find the Olympic National Forest and Mt Rainier National Park.

Paul Stamets, a mycologist, and entrepreneur, has his business, Fungi Perfecti, located in the Olympia area. This offers medicinal mushroom extracts and capsules to grow your own fungi.

It is important to control how many wild mushrooms you consume. Despite thoroughly cleaning and rinsing them, tiny toxins will still be present as they have been growing in the woods for a long time. Make sure to wash and cook them thoroughly before serving them.

Kennett Square, Pennsylvania

Kennett Square in Pennsylvania houses some of the United States' best and tastiest mushroom species. Local mushroom foraging experts and gourmet wild mushroom chefs give you cooking demonstrations on how to use your pickings in the best way possible. This place also has a quirky mushroom museum which exhibits the mushroom life cycle.

Chester County, Pennsylvania

Known for its sixty-one mushroom farms, Chester County is solely responsible for over four hundred million pounds of mushrooms in the United States, which are estimated to be valued at $365 million.

Around 47% of the country's mushrooms come from Chester County. Mushrooms are grown in barns, houses, and doubles.

The bulk of the mushrooms produced here belong to the Agaricus species. They are small white and brown button-like mushrooms and large portobellos, which are a popular side for steak. Apart from these mushrooms, the state is also an important source of "specialties" or "exotics" such as oysters, shiitakes, maitakes, beeches, etc.

There are many more places you can go foraging your heart out once you have learned the lay of the land. The trick is in opening your heart and mind and embracing your newfound love for mushroom foraging. The more you open your heart and mind, the more places you will discover, and the more fun you will have. One of the best parts of mushroom foraging is that you will build an extensive social circle across the globe as it becomes very easy to connect with like-minded people, thanks to the multiple social media platforms available at your fingertips.

Chapter Twelve

Debunking Mushroom Myths and Reinforcing Facts about Mushrooms

A mushroom hunt is something anyone would enjoy. Their electric gold and orange hues really bring life to the area surrounding them. They can be enjoyed in a variety of ways. They can be eaten with toast, garlic, parmesan, and many other things. However, there are many rumors which are centered around wild mushrooms, which say that it is best not to consume them. Others say that it is safe to eat mushrooms which smell good. This is not true. This article will try and clear common doubts which most mushroom hunters will have.

Are Mushrooms Plants?

Most people spend their lives believing mushrooms are plants. Mushrooms are even considered to be a part of a vegetarian diet. However, research shows that the genetics of mushrooms are more closely related to animals rather than plants. These genetic results show relationships between fungi and animals, which were prevalent more than 1.1 billion years ago. It is believed that the same single-celled organism gave birth to animals as well as a fungus, but it is hard to confirm this.

In conclusion, mushrooms don't belong to either the plant or animal kingdoms but a kingdom of their own.

Are Mushrooms Vegetables?

We know that mushrooms are not plants and are, therefore, definitely not vegetables. Mushrooms are actually born from fungi. They can be thought of as apples that originate from apple trees.

Are Mushrooms Consumed Only By Humans?

No, humans aren't the only species that consume mushrooms. In fact, research shows that mushrooms are a main source of food for creatures and insects which thrive in the deciduous and coniferous forests. They are also popular among squirrels.

They also contribute to the ecosystem by consuming the dead and decaying matter surrounding them. They can grow out of dead plants, trees, and even animals. They also form symbiotic relationships with other living animals as they have common nutrient needs with their host, including sugar, nitrogen, phosphorus, potassium, etc. They essentially eat their home.

Is Chanterelle the Only Edible Mushroom?

Chanterelle mushrooms are one of the many delicious mushrooms. Hedgehog mushrooms are also very popular to make mushroom broths. King Bolete, also known as France's Cèpe and Italy's porcini, is also very popular for its flavor.

Do Mushrooms Cause Candida?

Candida is a fungal infection that affects our skin and mucous membranes. Mushrooms are often associated with Candida due to its fungal origin. In fact, shiitake, an exotic mushroom variety famous in Japan, can fight against Candida. Shiitake works brilliantly by attacking only the pathogens without affecting the internal organs, thereby ensuring Candida is eliminated out of the affected person's system and keeping the side-effects almost negligible.

Can Mushrooms Build the Strength of the Immune System?

In symbiotic relationships, the mushrooms can impact the immune system of the host positively. Mushrooms tend to take certain nutrients from their hosts, and in return, give them the nutrients. For example, if the host's immune system has a problem, then a mushroom variety that lives in a symbiotic relationship with this host could pass on certain nutrients and minerals that could have an immunity-boosting effect.

Are All Mushrooms the Same?

There are many variations among different mushrooms species. They differ on where they are grown, under what conditions they are grown, whether they are organic or not, how they are extracted, what part of the mushroom is edible, etc.

Are Mushrooms Poisonous?

Among a large variety of fungi, some mushrooms are poisonous and can have very painful side effects, and there are some with powerful medicinal properties. It all really depends on how you choose your mushrooms and how confident and thorough you are on your mushroom research.

Cleaning Mushrooms Before Consuming Them is a Must

Mushrooms are moisture-loving organisms. While they grow outside, they absorb a lot of moisture for their survival. If you wash mushrooms again before cooking, they will release the excess water while you are cooking them and make your dish slimy. So, a quick rinse is the best way to wash mushrooms in order to clean them. Sometimes, using a brush to get rid of grit can work very well. A damp cloth can also be good enough. However, soaking mushrooms in water can be counterproductive in creating great mushroom dishes.

Are Wild Mushrooms Easy to Identify?

Most people identify wild and poisonous mushrooms by their spotted appearance. This is not enough. Many wild mushrooms do not have a spotted appearance. It is important to research what kind of mushroom you are looking for before you go into the woods on a mushroom hunt. Talk to a mushroom expert to sharpen what you already know about mushrooms.

Mushrooms Love to Grow in Dark, Underground Environments

Most mushrooms grow on the surface, next to a moist tree or dead and decaying matter. Mushrooms that grow underground are referred to as truffles, and they are one of the most expensive foods in the market.

Mushrooms Have no Nutritional Value Since They are Mostly Composed of Water

Even though about ninety percent of a mushroom is just water, they do contain a lot of minerals and vitamins, which are essential for the human body. They are rich in vitamin A and B complex. They are low in fat and are rich in protein.

Some Important Facts

Use Reliable and Verifiable Sources to Identify Your Mushrooms

Hunting for mushrooms without reliable information on how to distinguish them has the potential to go incredibly wrong. The 'Destroying Angel' bears a resemblance to many edible and delicious mushrooms that can actually lead to fatality when consumed. It's beautiful to look at so instinctively; one would go and pluck it and make the mistake of including it in their dish. These are capable of ruining your day, liver, or, worse, kill you too.

Sending a simple picture of a mushroom to a friend and getting their approval will not suffice. Many mushrooms look very similar to each other on the outside but are entirely different inside. You must delve deeper and speak to experts and take their opinion.

Mushroom Hunting Can be Done In A Team

Going mushroom hunting with your friend during the weekend can be a very fun activity. It is very easy to find mushroom communities who will always lend a helping hand. Moreover, you can always approach a mushroom expert to get your questions answered.

Do Not Overuse Your Mushroom Produce

Mushroom patches are very difficult to produce, and it is a slow procedure. Over-picking mushrooms can affect the next produce and even the creatures surrounding it. Take it slow and pick out only the amount of mushrooms which you need at that moment.

Some Interesting Facts About Mushrooms

France was one of the first countries to start growing mushrooms. Within a few years, the cultivation practice grew to England and is now prevalent even in the United States. There are around 10000 different species of mushrooms, out of which only 250 are known to be edible. Since mushrooms have no chlorophyll, they get their nutrients from other living trees and dead and decaying matter.

A mature mushroom is capable of dropping as many as sixteen billion spores.

Just one serving of button mushrooms (about five button mushrooms) has only twenty calories and constitutes no fat. They are, however, very rich in the vitamin B complex.

If you are lucky during one of your mushroom hunts in dense forests, you may come across a mushroom called Laetiporus, which tastes like fried chicken.

Ancient Egyptians believed that mushrooms were a vegetable that granted immortality.

It is believed that Viking invaders would consume hallucinogenic mushrooms to contain their rage. This was equivalent to today's alcohol.

The Fly Agaric mushroom, which looks very similar to the mushrooms in the Super Mario game does something similar to the mushroom in Super Mario. If consumed, the person will be under the illusion that all objects around them are larger than they actually are.

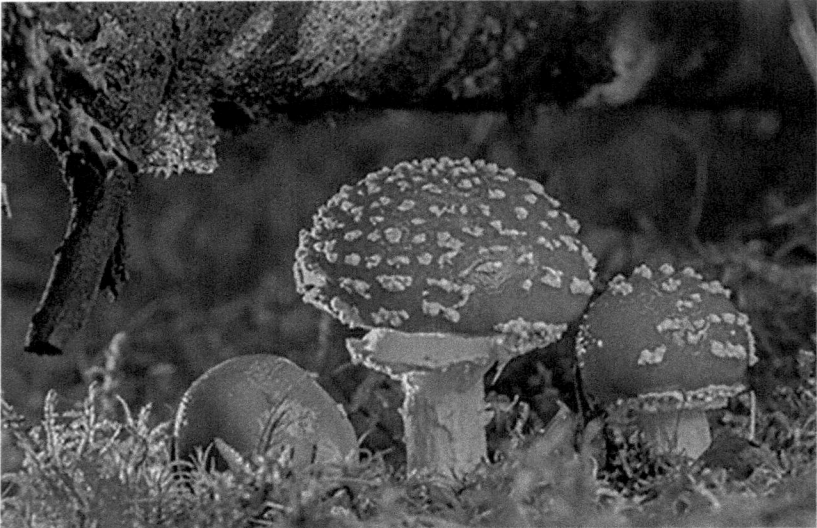

There is a poisonous mushroom that looks like a brain. It looks so poisonous that countries like Switzerland and Germany prohibit it from being sold.

Mushrooms tend to take on a very common circular pattern to grow in. This pattern is commonly referred to as the 'fairy ring.'

There is a mushroom which digests itself. The process can be very rapid, so it is recommended that this mushroom is cooked and eaten minutes after it is plucked.

Magic mushrooms are known for their alcohol-like after effects. However, some countries find it perfectly legal for people to purchase the spores of these mushrooms and breed them themselves.

Chapter Thirteen

How to Harvest Mushrooms
Ethically and Safely

The phrase 'ethical foraging' describes the rules and guidelines that foragers are bound to follow to prevent adverse effects on the environment and natural surroundings. The guidelines were framed from the lessons learned based on the outcomes of unwitting or unwitting mistakes made by earlier forgers.

The guidelines collected under the term of ethical foraging are designed to protect:

- The owners of the property on which foraging takes place.

- The foragers themselves.

- The environment and natural surroundings.

The three most important ethics based on conventional wisdom to follow unfailingly while picking and harvesting wild mushrooms are:

Do Not Over-Pick

While it may be true that over-picking mushrooms will not harm the underground mycelium, even then, it is a courteous and sensitive attitude not to pick more than what you need. An experienced picker learns the importance of picking not more than a third of what he or she sees and leaving the rest behind for the next picker who might come there. If all foragers practiced this rule of thumb, then there would be ample for everyone. Also, the mycelium has enough left to continue flourishing and fruiting for the next season.

A corollary of the over-picking point is to remind yourself that you are not a commercial mushroom gatherer. We are all recreational mushroom hunters, and we should pick up just enough for ourselves, and maybe to share with a few friends and family. Commercial hunting is all about focusing only on harvesting and nothing else. Commercial hunters can mercilessly get tons of mushrooms worth a lot of money picked in an incredibly short time. We are not this set.

Moreover, the permits that are given by forest officials often have the number of mushrooms you are allowed to pick, especially the rare and exotic ones. Sticking to the limit authorized by these permits is not only legally but also ethically good for you.

Also, when you pick mushrooms, be artful and graceful about it. You can gently pry or cut the mushrooms using a knife. Experts believe that as long as you are gentle with the way you pick your mushrooms, the future growth potential of the mycelium remains safe and intact.

Another crucial element to remember on this point is not to pick the last plant of any species ensuring you give a chance for the mushrooms to replenish and grow again.

Walk Gently on the Foraging Path

Tread gently on the path so that you don't trample and damage potential mushrooms under your feet. Hiking boots and other hard footwear that leave markings on the ground are not great for mushroom foraging. Moreover, keeping the trails, you find a secret from other foragers is part of the foraging deal among the experienced, the reason why experts will give you a general idea of where to go foraging but will never give away their secret hunting grounds.

Spreading Spores is a Good Forager's Responsibility

Spores are essentially seeds of the mushrooms that need to be released everywhere on the forest floor so that new mycelium and mushrooms can continue to flourish in the future. Here are some tips through which you can ensure you can do your duty to mushrooms spores:

Wherever and whenever possible, try and pick mature mushrooms whose spores are already released into the environment.

For those mushrooms that still have spores on them, make sure you use a wicker basket or any porous/holed container to put your pickings so that spores get dropped as you walk on your forest trail. Using plastic bags is the worst thing you can do when you go foraging for mushrooms. Here are some more ideas to ensure you harvest ethically:

While it is easy to make sure you don't leave behind large trash, it is also important to take care of the micro trash you could generate in your foraging trail. You mustn't leave any trash behind. Carry them with you and dispose of them responsibly.

More Tips for Safe and Ethical Harvesting of Mushrooms

Don't leave all the mushroom trimmings in the same place as you harvested them. Spread them around because these trimmings also have the potential to sprout new mycelium.

Also, look at mushrooms with a deep sense of curiosity. Leave behind and mark those places where you find unusual and unique mushrooms. Come back to the place on your next trip and see what has happened in the area. This approach is one of the best ways to learn about the life cycle of specific mushrooms. Understanding how harvesting and picking mushrooms affect their life cycle will help you build sustainability in mushroom foraging. You don't want to have excessive mushrooms in one season and nothing left to forage in the next season, right?

From the point of view of safety, you must learn to distinguish between edible and toxic and overly mature mushrooms. Also, when you see undesirable ones untouched, especially the overly mature and edible in their early stage, leave them so that they get to complete their life cycle. This way, you can get an opportunity to come back in time to pick the young ones the next time, or at least some other picker will have the opportunity to do so.

Follow the laws of the land and area you are foraging in. You must follow the approved maps of the region and ensure you don't trespass on forbidden and private property.

Some places have strict rules on the number of mushrooms allowed to be picked by foragers, and sticking to these laws is imperative. Moreover, some places could have a ban on commercial harvesting. Therefore, learn and follow the laws of the area. Nearly all foraging sites have bylaws that can be researched for and read online before starting off on your foraging expedition.

Some areas could have an extra-strict rule regarding endangered species of mushrooms. The endangering could be a result of over-harvesting or due to weather and other climate conditions. Know and learn about these endangered species and be sure to follow the rules that govern the picking of such mushrooms. You can find the endangered lists of specific areas in documents of departments that manage wildlife and agriculture. Expert foragers in these specific areas would also be sources of encyclopedic information.

Get a clear idea of which types of mushrooms grow in the region you are foraging. Learn about the best places to look for and where an abundance can be found. It is best to leave those mushrooms that are not growing in abundance because it is clear that they are struggling to reproduce. So, by leaving them alone, you are empowering their struggle for survival.

Local farmers and experts can be of excellent help when it comes to giving you information about which mushrooms grow in abundance and which of them are struggling to survive. As a beginner, you must learn to respect the knowledge of the local guides, hunters, and farmers if you want to notch up your knowledge and skill levels of mushroom foraging.

Checking for the toxicity of the soil and the environment is an important aspect to check for before beginning mushroom foraging. You should check out the area's topography to find out if it has been exposed to toxic chemicals of any kind. For example, if there is a chemical or fertilizer factory close by, you might want to check up on whether the effluents from there are affecting the soil in the region.

The toxins from the factory may be finding their way into the plants and trees in the surroundings. While there are strict laws to prevent such occurrences, as a beginner, it might be a good idea to use these ideas as valuable lessons, especially while identifying avoidable mushroom varieties. The local municipal offices and other government agencies allocated to monitor such things will help you out with the requisite data.

Learn to identify mushrooms based on more than one characteristic. When you have chosen a foraging destination, read up about the place, and gather information on 2-3 common mushroom species, you are likely to find there. Spend time to recognize and identify the features of these 2-3 species.

When you are thorough about these, then only move on to the next couple of species. This approach will help you learn about each type of mushroom theoretically first, and then apply your knowledge practically as you forage for mushrooms. This combination of theory and practice will build your mushroom foraging skills excellently.

And finally, remember to be a steward of nature. Careless and thoughtless harvesting reflects an attitude of callousness towards nature. An ethical forager respects and values Mother Nature.

Chapter Fourteen

Poisonous Mushroom in North America

N ote of caution: Many mushrooms look very similar and can be difficult to tell apart. Some can be deadly. If you are unsure, don't eat them!

The deadliest mushrooms known to man belong to genera (plural of genus) Amanita. The mushrooms of the Amanita genus account for a small percentage of all the mushroom species. However, this genus has some of the deadliest and most toxic mushroom species known to man.

The death cap or Amanita phalloides is believed to be the culprit in more than 90% fatalities caused by mushroom poisoning. One of the primary reasons for this is the fact that the death cap looks extremely appetizing and meaty. Another interesting statistic with regard to mushroom poisoning is a large percentage of East Asian and Southeast Asian immigrants have been victims. Experts attribute this large count to the similarities between the death cap and the paddy straw mushroom, a common variety found in Southeast and East Asian regions.

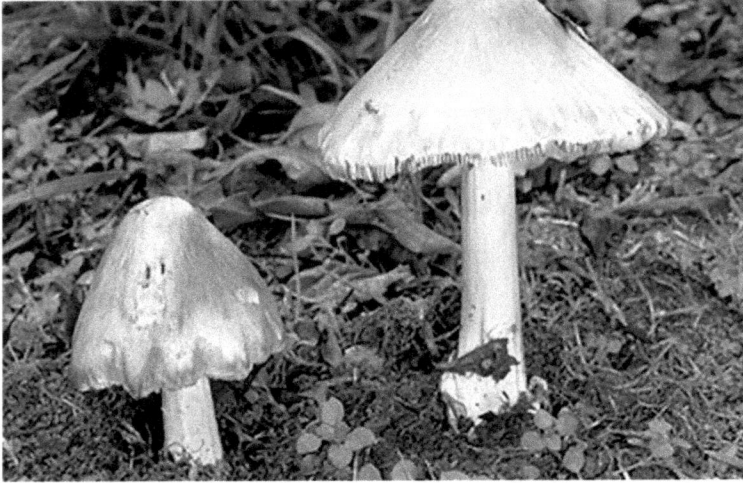

Death Cap Mushroom – Do NOT eat!

Interestingly, the genera Amanita also contains some of the most beautiful and tasty, edible mushroom species as well. For example, Amanita caesera, with its gorgeous orange-red profile, was a favorite of Roman Emperors as well as the ancient royal Egyptians.

The young, immature Amanitas are easily distinguishable by the universal veil-like cocoon that covers them. This also makes them look dangerously similar to puffball mushrooms. Most of the Amanita species have a collar-like volva at the base, which is another trademark characteristic of this genera.

Deadliest Known Mushrooms

Some common features that you can use to identify a few common poisonous mushrooms found in North America are:

Amanita phalloides

Known as death caps, the biological name of this deadly mushroom variety is Amanita phalloides. Experts give it the first rank when it comes to fatality count in the number of global mushroom poisoning cases.

Incidentally, this variety of mushroom is believed to have been brought into North America accidentally, perhaps along with tree imports from Europe. But, they have now spread all over the continent even though they are not very common. Native to Europe, death caps are found in many parts of the US Eastern and Western Coasts.

Death caps feature 6-inch yellow, brown, green, or white caps that are often sticky to the touch. The stalks of these poisonous mushrooms are usually 5 inches tall and grow on white-colored cup-like bases under oaks, dogwoods, pines, and other such trees.

Normally seen from September to November, death caps can be easily mistaken for puffball mushrooms of genera Lycoperdon, Calbovista, and Calvatia. The deadliest aspect of death caps is that there are no immediate worry-causing symptoms. After a while, the person is likely to experience vomiting, cramps, and diarrhea, which also disappear after a few days, which makes people think that they are fine.

Unfortunately, during this 'okay' time, the poison of death caps would be damaging all the internal organs, many times irreversible. Death is known to occur between 6 to 18 days after consumption. The most prominent toxin in the Death Cap is known as a-amanitin. The potency of this toxin is not eliminated or even reduced by any cooking method or freezing.

The young Death Cap is often mistaken for the edible Wood Mushroom and Field Mushroom, both of the Agaricus genera. Also, the Death Cap mushroom in its button stage can be mistaken for the non-poisonous and edible puffballs. Interestingly, squirrels and rabbits are not affected by this poisonous mushroom, and therefore, checking to see if wild animals eat it before you pick them is an extremely bad idea to discern between poisonous and non-poisonous varieties.

Here are some vital identification marks for the Death Cap:

- The caps (ranging between 5 and 15 cm in diameter) of the Death Cap are almost pure white at the immature stage, and as they mature, the color of the caps changes to yellow, olive, or bronze, with the center nearly becoming black.

- Initially, the caps are egg-shaped. As they mature, the caps become almost flat. A decaying death cap gives off an extremely unpleasant odor.

- The stem of the death cap grows to a height of 7 to 15 cm. They are off-white in color and look paler than the cap and have zig-zag mottling.

- The gills are broad and free and white initially. As the mushroom matures, the gills become cream-colored. Sometimes, the gills get a slight pinkish tinge as the body ages.

- The base of the Death Cap is swollen and surrounded by a large, sack-like volva with a greenish-color inside.

- The spores of the Death Cap are white, and the shape ranges from ellipsoidal to subglobose.

The non-poisonous look-alike mushrooms of the Agaricus genera do not have a volva. Also, the gills of the immature edible variety are gray or pinkish-brown, which is not the case with the gills of the Death Cap is pure white at the immature stage.

Another important point to ensure you are not picking an Amanita mistaking it to be an Agaricus is this; the volva of the Amanita might have broken or remained hidden underground. So, to be sure, it makes sense to dig up the soil and look for the broken or hidden volva before consuming it.

Amanita bisporigera and Amanita ocreata

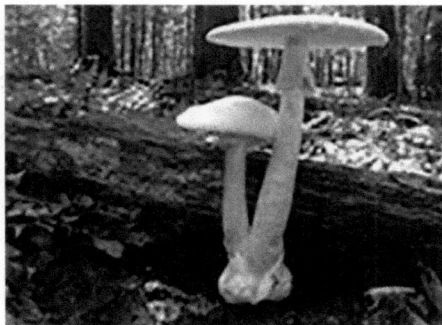

Do NOT eat!

Belonging to the genus Amanita, these deadly mushrooms (also referred to as death angels or destroying angels) are called angels because all the species have pure white caps and stalks. Their white stalks, caps, and gills are almost beautiful to look at, and it is easy to get attracted to these mushrooms. Their innocuous lookalikes include horse mushrooms, meadow mushrooms, button mushrooms, and puffballs.

Destroying angels are widely seen across the US during the summer and fall seasons. These mushrooms connect themselves to the roots of certain trees, plants, and shrubs. You can see them growing in and near the woodlands and also in suburban laws.

The symptoms of poisoning by consuming destroying angels include abdominal pain, diarrhea, and nausea, which usually set in within 5 to 12 hours after ingestion. These symptoms also tend to go away for a while, making the person think that he or she is alright. However, the symptoms will return a couple of days and with a vengeance.

Sadly, when the symptoms return, it might be too late to do anything as many of the internal organs, including kidney and liver, would have been damaged irreversibly. Typically, people affected by the poison of destroying angels tend to end up in a fatal hepatic coma.

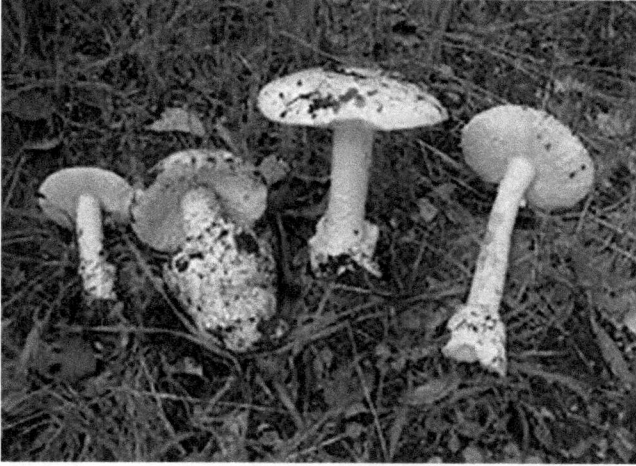

Do NOT eat!

Amanita muscaria

Referred to as the Fly Agaric, Amanita muscaria is a hallucinogen and commonly found in many of the woodlands in the northern hemisphere, including the USA and Canada, and the British Isles. The name Fly Agaric was given to it because traditionally, the mushroom was used as an insecticide. There are many varieties of Amanita muscaria, including:

- Amanita muscaria var. formosa - is a familiar sight in North America with its orange-yellow or yellow cap, a yellow stem, and covered in yellow spots.

- Amanita muscaria var. alb - is a white form of the Fly Agaric, which is a rare mushroom.

- Amanita muscaria var. regalis - is a brown form of the Fly Agaric. Some experts treat this as a separate species and refer to it as Amanita regalis.

The toxins present in this mushroom have different symptoms in different people and also based on the quantity consumed. For example, consuming dried form of Fly Agaric can cause nausea, drowsiness, sweating, euphoria, dizziness, and distortions in sounds and sights. Experts believe that the toxins in these mushrooms are psychoactive compounds, too, which have various hallucinogenic effects.

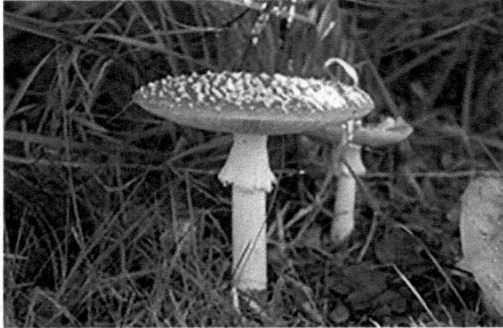

Do NOT eat!

The hallucinogenic effects are believed to have been in use since time immemorial. They may even be humankind's oldest known hallucinogen. Experts believe that Amanita muscaria was used extensively around the globe right from the early Indian civilizations to the Viking invaders to the more contemporary Siberian shamans.

The mushrooms of the Amanita muscaria species are fatal when consumed in large quantities. Hence, reported deaths from this species are fewer in number as compared to that of the other poisonous varieties.

In North America, Amanita muscaria var. Formosa which is referred to as Amanita muscaria var. Guessowii. Some of the characteristic features of this variety of this mushroom found in North America are:

This mushroom is widely distributed in northeast parts of North America and in the northern Midwest.

- The cap ranges between 5 and 19 cm in diameter. It is round at the center and becomes increasingly convex and almost flat at the edges.

- The color of the cap could range from pale yellow to bright yellow, orange-yellow to reddish-yellow. These colors tend to fade with age.

- The caps have cottony warts, the color of which could be whitish or yellowish. These patches are sticky when fresh.

- The gills are very loosely attached to the stem, and sometimes even free from it. Gills are usually found only in the marginal areas.

- Ranging from a length of 6 to 30 cm and between 1 and 3.5 cm in thickness, the stems of this species of North American mushrooms have a wide base and a tapering apex.

- The flesh of this mushroom remains white throughout its lifetime, even when it is sliced or cut.

Galerina marginata

Commonly known as Funeral Bell, the toxins found in Galerina marginata are similar to those found in death caps or Amanita phalloides. These deadly mushrooms are commonly found all across North America, including the United States. They are found in Europe, Russia, Japan, and many other Asian regions as well.

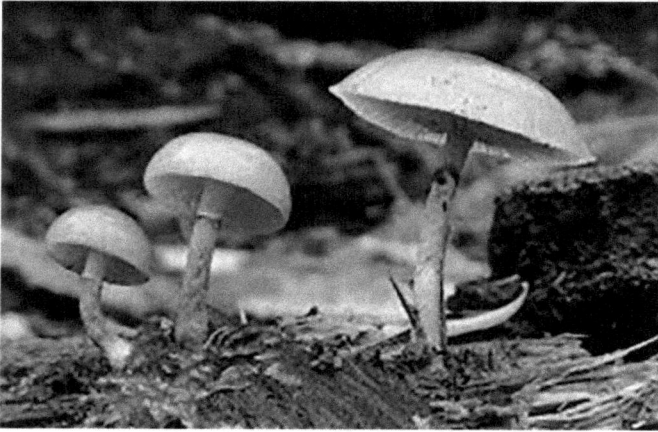

Do NOT eat!

With broad, brown caps and thin stems, these deadly mushrooms cause severe gastrointestinal problems, which, if left untreated, result in liver failure leading to coma, and eventually, death.

The notorious Funeral Bell can be found on the stumps, fallen branches, and dead tree trunks of conifers as well as on the stumps of a few broadleaf trees. The Funeral Bell can easily be confused with the edible mushroom called Wood Tuft or Brown Stew Fungus.

One of the reasons why the Funeral Bell has not caused as many deaths as the death cap is because its innocuous edible lookalike, Wood Tuft, is not a much sought-after mushroom variety. Also, the Funeral Bell is not as commonly occurring as the Death Caps.

Here are Some Tips for Identifying the Funeral Bell

- The cap of the Funeral Bell is hemispherical initially and slowly tapers off into a broad convex or nearly flat shape. The caps are brown in the middle and fade to a light honey-yellow color at the edges. The cap's diameter ranges between 1 to 7 cm.

- The stem of the Funeral Bell ranges between 2 to 7 cm in length and 2 to 7 mm in diameter. The apex of the stem is usually buff-colored and becomes browner towards the base.

- The color of the gills ranges from the honey-colored to a pale cream-fawn and takes on a slightly rusty color as the mushrooms mature. The spores of the Funeral Bell are elliptical in shape and have a snuff brown color.

- The Funeral Bell has a mealy smell

The Brown Stew Fungus, the edible lookalike, is similar in color and size. However, the cap of the edible mushroom has a pale-colored center and dark rims and are found mostly on hardwood substrates. Most importantly, the Brown Stew Fungus does not have a meaty odor.

False Morels

False morels are a group of mushrooms that bear an uncanny resemblance to the highly popular and famous morel mushrooms. Mushrooms of the Gyromitra genus are usually referred to as false morels. Novice mushroom foragers can easily mistake false morels for being the edible ones. However, with a bit of experience, this learning gap can be quickly covered, and discerning between false morels and edible ones becomes easy.

Gyromitra esculenta - This species is most commonly referred to as "false morels." It has numerous common names, including beefsteak mushroom, brain mushroom, elephant ears, and turban mushrooms. All these names refer to this variety's convoluted, wrinkled shape.

It is one of the most toxic false morels and also bears a striking and easily mistakable resemblance to the edible morels. Some of the distinguishing characteristic features of the highly toxic Gyromitra esculenta are:

- These false morels usually grow under conifers.

- The convoluted-shaped cap of this mushroom species has multiple folds and wrinkles.

- The color of the cap can be pinkish, reddish-brown, or almost black, depending on the maturity of the mushroom.

- The underside of the cap is almost always invisible.

- The interior of the cap is partially hollow, and the fleshy parts are of a tan color.

- This false morel does not have any gills.

- Reddish to orangish spores is produced and found on the surface of the cap.

- The stem is thin and short and has deep, vertical folds and pale in color. The stem is never hollow. True morels have hollow stems.

Interestingly, the toxins in Gyromitra esculenta can be eliminated by cooking the mushrooms. However, the fumes emanating from the cooking vessel are also toxic. Moreover, the amount of toxins in each mushroom is highly variable. So, you can never be sure if you have removed all the toxins by cooking.

Sometimes, toxins are fully removed, making the cooked mushroom edible, whereas, sometimes, there could be toxins enough to kill still remaining after the cooking process. So, it is best not to attempt cooking or to eat false morels. This information is just that, information only.

Gyromitra caroliniana - Like the Gyromitra esculenta, the cap of this mushroom species is highly wrinkled and has a distinctive red color. The stem of this species is quite thick, especially at the base. It is found near rotting logs and stumps of hardwood trees and is a common sight during spring in southeastern parts of North America.

Omphalotus olearius

Omphalotus olearius, commonly referred to as Jack O' Lantern mushrooms closely resemble chanterelles, one of the most prized edible mushrooms on earth. Chanterelles are meaty and delicious and are found in plenty under conifers and hardwoods. Jack O' Lanterns are bioluminescent mushrooms that clear and decompose and live off wood debris in hardwood forests.

The seasonal fruiting patterns and the famous and distinguishing orange colors of Jack O' Lanterns closely match with chanterelles. However, while chanterelles are delectable and much sought-after, Jack O' Lanterns are poisonous. They contain the toxin muscarine, which causes multiple gastrointestinal problems, including severe diarrhea and stomach cramps. Although this mushroom does not result in a fatality, hospitalization is almost a certainty. So, it is best to avoid consuming the Jack O' Lantern.

The biggest attraction towards this toxic mushroom is its close resemblance to a much sought-after gourmet mushroom, the chanterelle. It is easy for beginners to be carried away by the excitement of believing they have found a chanterelle when, in reality, they could be holding the toxic Jack O' Lantern.

Therefore, you must rein in your excitement and do a thorough examination before consuming any mushroom. In fact, as a beginner, the wisest thing you can do is to show all the mushrooms you have picked to an expert for a second opinion before cooking or consuming them. Here are some facts about this interesting but inedible mushroom:

- The cap and stem of the mushroom are colored from bright orange to greenish orange.

- Initially, the cap is smooth and is convex or flat. As the mushrooms mature, the caps turn upwards.

- The stem is also smooth to touch.

- There is sac at the base or ring on top of the stem.

- This saprophytic mushroom tends to grow on dead hardwoods, especially oak trees.

- You can see Jack O' Lanterns from late summer into fall.

- Another attractive feature of this toxic variety is its bioluminescence, which means they glow in the dark, thanks to a special enzyme they have in their body.

The debate about the name of the exact species found in North America still rages on. Some experts think the North American species is actually Omphalotus illudens (which grows on the east coast) and Omphalotus olivascens (which grows on the west coast). Regardless of the name, the poisonous effects and their appearance are similar. It is best not to pick those mushrooms that match the identification marks mentioned above.

It is important to learn to distinguish between gourmet chanterelles and Jack O' Lanterns. The most important difference can be seen when you look at the gills. The gills of chanterelles are false gills that cannot be ripped off easily from under the cap. They are folded or wrinkled inwards. The gills of Jack O' Lanterns are non-forked, sharp, and can be picked off from under the cap, although a lot of care is needed considering the knife-like gills can cut your skin.

Conclusion

The concluding chapter in this book is a summarized list of the top tips that will help any beginner get a fabulous kick start to one of the most exciting hobbies, namely mushroom foraging. So, here is a list of your must-have tips for use during mushroom foraging. Don't forget to learn them by rote. You will thank yourself for doing it.

When on a Foraging Hunt, Focus on the Ground

The forest takes on a new perspective when you choose to focus on the forest floor. You will begin to notice innumerable flora, fauna, insects, and many tiny life forms that you didn't even know existed until you focused on the forest floor. As a non-forager, you would be accustomed to seeing and enjoying aerial views of verdant, thick forests, and wildlife. This focus has to change when you are foraging for mushrooms. Look down instead of up when foraging for mushrooms.

Birch and Beech Trees are Excellent Homes for Many Mushrooms

Mushrooms seem to love the vicinity of birch and beech trees, especially among mulch leaves. Piles of dead wood around these two types of trees are excellent places to begin your search.

Use the Help of Experts and Experienced Foragers

Both these categories of people love to share their knowledge about mushrooms. Your first foraging expedition should ideally be in the company of an expert. You can watch and learn from such people. Moreover, their excitement when they locate a rare or exotic mushroom is infectious, and your passion for the activity will go up a few notches.

If you cannot find an expert, then you can join an organized tour of mushroom foraging. These tours are regularly conducted by foraging clubs and groups. Alternatively, you can do your own research and go to a particular forest or countryside. You are likely to find many organized foraging tours by the local experts in the area, many times in conjunction with regulatory authorities. This means all the permits and other regulatory needs would be taken care of by experienced experts, and you can simply focus on the joy and learning from the foraging expedition.

Take an Offline or Online Mushroom Guide Book with Pictures

As you find your mushrooms, using pictures from offline or online guide books, reference books is a great way to check out your findings before harvesting them. This approach will not only help you keep away from poisonous and inedible varieties but also help you bridge theory and practice. While online resources are great, it might be a good idea to remind yourself that internet coverage in forest areas may not be very good.

Don't forget to show your gratitude to Mother Nature by ensuring you follow ethical and safe mushroom foraging processes. Mother Nature has enough for everyone's need but nothing for anyone's greed.

And finally, the best tip you can get from any mushroom forager book is this (even if it has been repeated a couple of times before):

"If in doubt, leave it out!" If you cannot identify a mushroom with 100% confidence, do not consume it. Nothing is more important than your life and health. And if these two elements are absent, then the excitement and fun in mushroom foraging have no value.

If you observe keenly, a large part of connecting with nature and restoring the balance of our ecosystem is based on nothing more than a little bit of common sense. Empower yourself with basic skills and then develop the beautiful art of mushroom foraging so that you can quickly, safely, and proudly move from a novice to an expert.

Mushroom foraging is one of the easiest hobbies to start off. All you need is wicker or any kind of porous basket, a decent pair of knives/scissors, and you are ready to go. Even if you don't get to pick the choicest of mushrooms in your initial foraging days, you can rest assured that you will feel the empowering benefits of this activity. It all starts with fun and excitement and goes right up to enhancing your physical, mental, and spiritual well-being.

Moreover, foraging areas are widely available all over North America, and the government agencies have thrown open these regions for recreational foragers. As long as you stick to the rules and regulations of the local area, you will be welcomed happily by most owners to forage in their property. Moreover, while the activity of foraging itself is physically beneficial, the health benefits from the collected mushrooms find their way into your kitchen, too, as you harness the multiple nutritional advantages of mushrooms grown naturally in the wild.

So, go on, and find your passion, and don't let the seemingly steep learning curves dampen your spirits. Be patient with yourself, and rest assured you will become an expert that other beginners would reach out to sooner than later.

References

https://www.alimentarium.org/en/knowledge/history-gathering-food

https://britishlocalfood.com/what-is-foraging/

https://www.healthista.com/13-reasons-to-be-outdoors-and-foraging-for-food/

https://www.moneycrashers.com/foraging-guide-edible-wild-plants-food/

https://www.goodhousekeeping.com/health/diet-nutrition/a27633487/mushroom-health-benefits/

https://food.ndtv.com/food-drinks/5-amazing-reasons-to-add-mushrooms-to-your-daily-meals-1705629

https://www.treehugger.com/wild-mushrooms-what-to-eat-what-to-avoid-4864324

http://mushroomwizard.com/_pages/_index_pages/n_a_deadly.html

https://www.first-nature.com/fungi/galerina-marginata.php

https://www.first-nature.com/fungi/amanita-phalloides.php

http://themushroomforager.com/2010/09/21/amanitas-from-deadly-to-delicious/

https://www.mushroomexpert.com/amanita_muscaria_guessowii.html

https://healing-mushrooms.net/gyromitra-esculenta

https://healing-mushrooms.net/false-morels

https://www.sceltamushrooms.com/en/themes/what-is-a-mushroom/

https://www.mushroom-appreciation.com/types-of-mushrooms.html#sthash.PpSGRnYj.dpbs

https://www.nytimes.com/wirecutter/blog/how-to-hunt-mushrooms/

https://1stchineseherbs.com/parts-of-mushrooms/

https://www.plantsnap.com/blog/edible-mushrooms-united-states/

https://www.mushroom-appreciation.com/drying-mushrooms.html#sthash.3zVSx0aH.dpbs

https://fungially.com/how-to-preserve-mushrooms-awesome-methods-to-know/

https://www.madaboutmushrooms.com/mad_about_mushrooms/2007/04/soups.html

http://mycowest.net/articles/p-9903jr.htm#:~:text=Advantages%20%2D%20Drying%20preserves%20mushrooms%20for,many%20species%2C%20especially%20the%20Boletes.

https://herbarium.usu.edu/fun-with-fungi/fairy-rings

https://foragerchef.com/fairy-ring-mushrooms-marasmius-oreades/

https://healing-mushrooms.net/marasmius-oreades

https://wildfoodism.com/2015/04/02/how-to-find-and-identify-morel-mushrooms/

http://mushroom-collecting.com/mushroomhedgehog.html

https://foragerchef.com/hedgehog-mushrooms/

https://foragerchef.com/in-a-yard-near-you-agaricus-campestrismeadow-mushroom/

https://honest-food.net/meadow-mushroom-recipe-escoffier/

https://healing-mushrooms.net/agaricus-campestris

https://foragerchef.com/the-shaggy-mane-mushroomlawyers-wig/

https://practicalselfreliance.com/shaggy-mane-mushrooms/

https://foragerchef.com/hen-of-the-woods-mushrooms/

http://tenrandomfacts.com/bears-head-tooth-fungus/

https://www.ediblewildfood.com/bears-head-tooth.aspx

https://specialtyproduce.com/produce/Bears_Head_Mushrooms_11322.php

https://practicalselfreliance.com/foraging-reishi-mushrooms/#:~:text=Ganoderma%20tsugae%20%E2%80%93%20Found%20in%20the,were%20growing%20close%20to%20hemlock.

https://www.ediblewildfood.com/reishi-mushroom.aspx

https://www.mushroom-appreciation.com/chicken-of-the-woods.html#sthash.DoGY2ZoI.dpbs

https://www.ediblewildfood.com/chicken-of-the-woods.aspx

https://www.cbc.ca/news/canada/newfoundland-labrador/andie-bulman-mushroom-pov-1.5644845

https://mushrooms4life.com/common-mushroom-myths/

https://www.walshmushrooms.com/Mushroom_Myths--post--177.html

https://recipes.howstuffworks.com/food-facts/mushroom-facts.htm

https://www.kickassfacts.com/25-kickass-interesting-facts-mushrooms/

https://www.mushroom-appreciation.com/black-trumpet.html#sthash.H02lY1AA.dpbs

http://foragedfoodie.blogspot.com/2018/09/identifying-black-trumpet-mushrooms.html

https://practicalselfreliance.com/foraging-and-using-chaga-mushroom/

https://foragerchef.com/puffball-mushrooms/

https://themushroomforager.com/category/giant-puffball/

http://www.thesurvivalgardener.com/how-to-identify-an-edible-bolete-mushroom/

https://forestorigins.com/blogs/mushroom-blog-posts/the-mushroom-life-cycle

https://www.mushroom-appreciation.com/omphalotus-olearius.html

https://www.modern-forager.com/sustainable-mushroom-picking/

https://www.herbal-supplement-resource.com/ethical-foraging/

https://ecosystemrestorationcamps.org/the-joys-of-mushroom-foraging-for-beginners/

https://www.wpr.org/5-wild-foods-forage-wisconsin-summer

https://scienceline.org/2019/03/foraging-with-new-york-citys-mushroom-hunters/

http://www.plantpath.cornell.edu/labs/hodge/MushroomClub.html

https://www.lonelyplanet.com/articles/best-us-foraging-spots

https://www.sparefoot.com/self-storage/blog/23676-the-5-best-u-s-cities-for-mushroom-foragers-to-move-to/

https://www.travelandleisure.com/food-drink/the-best-places-in-the-world-to-travel-if-you-love-mushrooms

https://modernfarmer.com/2014/05/welcome-mushroom-country-population-nearly-half-u-s-mushrooms/

https://www.argobuilder.com/wisconsin-mushroom-hunting.html

http://everintransit.com/hunting-mushrooms-on-the-california-coast-and-living-to-tell-the-tale/

https://www.forestmushrooms.com/pages/black-trumpet-recipes

https://chaga101.com/chaga-recipes/

http://www.appalachianfeet.com/2010/12/03/how-to-find-
hedgehog-mushrooms-and-eat-them-with-recipes/

https://foragerchef.com/classic-fried-puffballs/

https://foragerchef.com/bolete-julienne/

https://honest-food.net/meadow-mushroom-recipe-escoffier/

https://foragerchef.com/parmesan-crusted-shaggy-manes/

http://littleindiana.com/2013/10/fried-sheepshead-mushrooms-
recipe/

https://foragerchef.com/wild-mushrooms-with-garlic-and-parsley/

https://www.cbc.ca/life/thegoods/reishi-mushroom-veggie-soup-
1.5032793

https://cdn.pixabay.com/photo/2014/07/10/20/55/mushroom-
389421__340.jpg

https://pixabay.com/photos/cep-dried-mushrooms-dried-
mushrooms-1719553/

https://pixabay.com/photos/mushrooms-morels-nature-edible-
1053367/

https://pixabay.com/photos/morel-mushroom-hose-mushroom-
smell-468690/

https://pixabay.com/photos/fungus-mushroom-sponge-basket-
1194380/

https://pixabay.com/photos/hexenring-mushroom-ring-feenring-4683784/

https://pixabay.com/photos/mushroom-meadow-mushroom-lamellar-3769313/

https://pixabay.com/photos/shaggy-mane-wild-mushroom-fungi-4564939/

https://pixabay.com/photos/giant-puffballs-calvatia-gigantea-185481/

https://pixabay.com/photos/cep-spruce-bolete-herrenpilz-4569397/

https://pixabay.com/photos/baumschwamm-reishi-770056/

https://pixabay.com/photos/sulphur-mushroom-2362179/

https://pixabay.com/photos/mushroom-black-trumpet-mushroom-175800/

https://cdn.pixabay.com/photo/2017/10/20/09/47/chaga-2870598__340.jpg

https://cdn.pixabay.com/photo/2017/10/04/21/36/fly-agaric-2817723__340.jpg

https://cdn.pixabay.com/photo/2019/11/21/20/35/mushroom-4643456__340.jpg

https://cdn.pixabay.com/photo/2017/01/06/12/36/fly-agaric-1957614__340.jpg

FORAGING

FOR BEGINNERS

*Identifying Medicinal Plants in
North America*

MONA GREENY

Introduction

Foraging has become one of the most popular hobbies and sustainable life choices in the past few years. The ability to forage wild plants and utilize them for either food or their medicinal properties is a skill that everyone should possess. The more plants you know about, the better your skills, and survival chances will be. Even the simplest Dandelion is packed with minerals, vitamins, and various medicinal properties. This book can help you learn how to identify a lot of wild herbs. It will also help you learn what health benefits these plants possess.

In this book, you will learn about the basics of foraging and a variety of medicinal plants. You will find out information regarding common herbs, how to use them, how to preserve them, etc. You will find simple but detailed instructions on how to recognize some of the most common wild herbs around North America and how to use them. The book will help you learn how to harness the power of nature for your benefit without harming it.

For the benefit of the reader, the various herbs and medicinal plants have been divided into multiple categories according to the region where they are found. This way, you will be able to check for an herb quickly without having to go through the whole book repeatedly.

A detailed chapter on various herbal products will help you understand how to use the herbs. Similarly, a detailed chapter on the basics of foraging will help the beginners to start their foraging journey with ample knowledge.

Foraging can be a wonderful experience with a lot of benefits. Just be careful about the plants that you pick, and you will surely be able to live a long and healthy life.

Chapter 1

Basics of Foraging

M ost of the wild plants and herbs listed in this book can be identified with ease, but certain plants will need more expertise. If you are an absolute beginner, it is necessary to study some of the more 'exotic' plants carefully so that you will be able to avoid accidents. If possible, get a local botanist or a wildcrafter to show you the difference between the plants. Do not pick a medicinal herb unless you are completely sure of its identity and species. Once you learn how to harvest a particular plant, chances are you will never forget how to do so in the future.

The herbs described in this book are beneficial in multiple ways, but it is recommended to check the herbs and their potency with a doctor before using them. Certain herbs can be dangerous if they are mixed with certain drugs. Similarly, some herbs can lead to catastrophic results if not used properly.

While consuming wild plants, our natural senses of smell, taste, and to a certain extent, sight can warn us of danger. Plants that consist high amount of tannin will always taste exceptionally discomforting.

Many toxic plants look like they are toxic. They often look scary or creepy. Generally, bright white and red colors tend to be poisonous (but not in all cases). Due to the inherent danger of consuming plants, it is always better to be safe and careful.

To begin your foraging journey, it is recommended to begin with the herbs that you already know and can identify. Read the chapter regarding the herb in this book and check how to harvest it and what medicinal properties it has. It is recommended to establish a foraging community with a bunch of like-minded people. The group should consist of enthusiasts, naturalists, herbalists, forestry experts, and botanists, along with photographers, etc.

Are Wild Plants Better?

Almost all the plants and herbs described here can be bought in bulk from the market or online. However, it is recommended to either grow or forage your plants instead of buying them. There is a multitude of reasons why you should forage wild plants instead of buying them. By foraging your plants, you will be aware of the source of your herbs, and you will be able to consume and use only the most potent and high-quality products. It is also a far more economical and viable option as compared to buying plants from the market.

The biggest reason why you should consider foraging over buying herbs from stores is freshness. Foraged herbs will always be fresher as compared to store-bought herbs. Store-bought herbs are often sprayed with chemicals or are waxed, heated, or coated with certain chemicals. They are also exposed to irradiation, refrigeration, exhaust, germs, and pesticides. Foraging cuts down all the processing and provides you fresh and 100% natural products. This will bring you much-needed peace of mind.

Ethical Wildcrafting

While foraging herbs and plants for medicinal and other purposes, it is necessary to keep certain things in mind. Certain herbs have gone mainstream, and now everyone wants to try them. This has led to over-harvesting, which has made the species threatened. Never over forage and only take absolutely necessary plants. Certain foraging methods are akin to pruning. This enhances the growth of the plant and does not threaten the species.

Whenever you harvest the flowering tops of plants, you should leave a lot of growth opportunities while making the cut. Never harvest all the flowers from a plant—the flowers produce seeds for propagation, and if you take all the flowers, the plant will not propagate. Whenever you dig a root or a tuber, plant a part of it in the ground again. This is sustainable foraging, which will prove beneficial for everyone.

The Best Time to Forage

A lot of herbs can be harvested almost any time of the year, but certain plants need to be harvested in specific seasons only. The best time to harvest leaves and flowers is when they are new and fresh. This changes according to the species and the plant as well. Check out the growth cycle of the plant before harvesting it. Pick the leaves just before the flowering starts. Pick flowers when they are new and look vibrant. Harvest roots at the beginning of fall or spring. Avoid harvesting the roots when the plant is in bloom or has leaves. Harvest the roots before the leaves come out or once they die away.

It is recommended to harvest leaves and flowers around 10 AM. On cloudy days the harvesting period is much longer. In most of the plants, once the flowers wilt, the leaves become bitter, and their potency goes down. Roots can be harvest at any time of the day.

Common Sense and Foraging

There are many different places where you can find herbs and plants. You can find them in woods, meadows, fields, grasses, etc. You can find many potent herbs in your backyard too.

Check the health of the land and the atmosphere before foraging plants. For instance, never harvest plants that are situated next to the roads.

If you plan to forage from someone else's property, please ask for permission lest you end up trespassing.

Chapter 2

Medical Plants of Meadows

Most of these plants are easily found in open areas, yards, roadsides, etc. and they can be grown in your garden as well.

Alfalfa Fabaceae

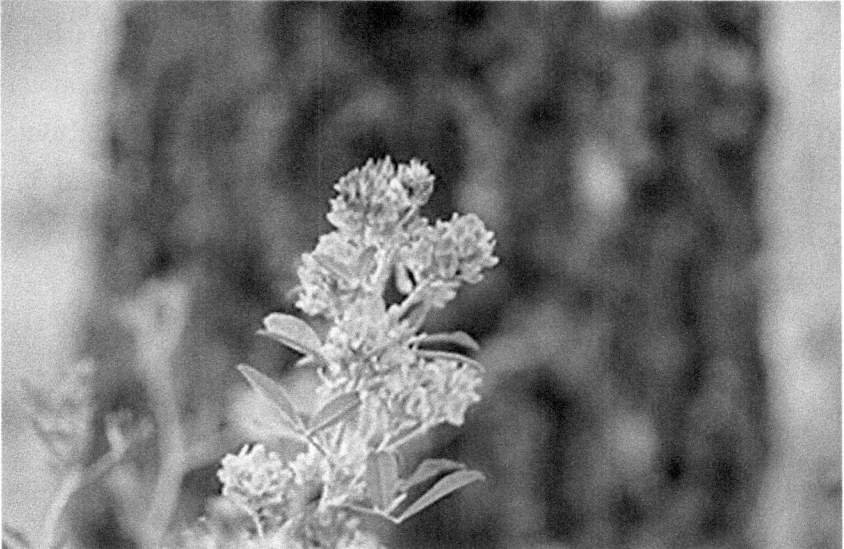

(Medicago sativa L.)

Identification

These are perennials with tiny, purple, or lavender colored flowers. They have a short raceme and generally have five petals and the plant grows around 20" to 4' tall. The stem is angular, erect, and smooth. The leaves are toothed in the front and have a sharp tip. Leaves are alternate.

Habitat

Found on lower alpine slopes, in fields, and pastures.

Uses

Fresh/dried leaves and sprouts can be used to improve digestion. It also alkalizes urine, which can detoxify the body. Alfalfa can also tackle excess cholesterol, inflammation, and fungus. It also improves anemic conditions and balance of the hormones. It is also used to treat ulcers, skin conditions, some colon problems, and can also strengthen bones and joints. Alfalfa has antimicrobial and antifungal properties. It also has cosmetic properties and is good for hair growth.

Caution

Alfalfa has virtually no side effects if it is cooked and consumed in moderation. Some people are allergic to alfalfa, and it can trigger lupus in people who are prone to it. Avoid eating seeds ass it may impair blood clotting in the long term. Children should avoid this.

Asiatic Dayflower

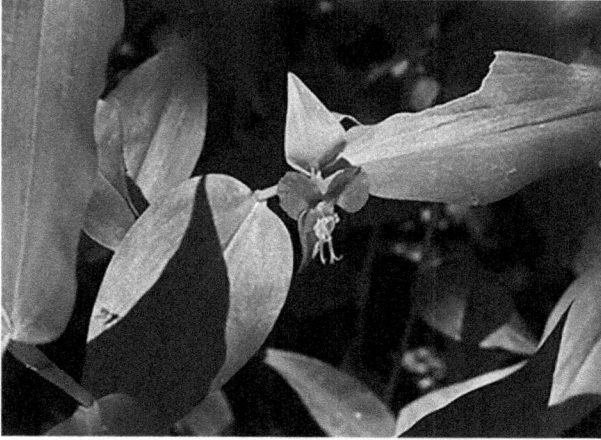

Commelinaceae (Commelina communis L.)

Identification

It is commonly found as a weed in many gardens. It has erect stems that collapse soon and deep blue flowers that look like Mickey's ears. Leaves are oblong and about 5" long with pointed tips. Are present in the form of a sheath around the stem.

Habitat

Easily found along roadsides and in the garden. (Originally from China.)

Edible

Leaves and flowers can be consumed in the form of teas.

Uses

It contains Phytosterols and isoflavones. Seeds contain nonessential and essential amino and fatty acids and the seedpods are edible.

Asparagus

Asparagaceae (Asparagus officinalis L.)

Identification

Asparagus is a perennial plant that can grow up to 60" tall. It has feathery foliage and fasciculated tubers. Flowers are greenish-yellowish and bloom singly or in clusters. Male and female flowers grow on different plants (generally). The fruit is red and is often poisonous for humans.

Habitat

It can be found along roadsides and fencerows and loves saline soil.

Food

It can be sautéed, steamed, roasted, etc. It is great with pizza, fish, beef, poultry, etc.

Harvest

Pick in spring before the feathery leaves start to grow.

Uses

Ancient practices believe that it can be used to treat gout, but modern medicine says that it can make the symptoms worse. In Spanish medicines, it is used to treat UTIs and kidney stones. According to certain scientific evidence, asparagus has anti-leukemia properties. It is a cleansing food that is good for the urinary tract. It has multiple micronutrients, which makes it great for the immunity power.

Dandelion

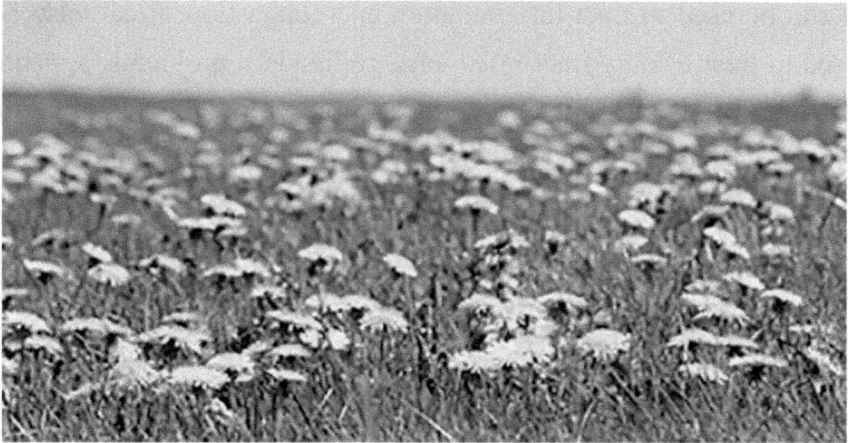

Asteraceae (Taraxacum officinale G.H. Weber ex Wiggers)

Identification

It is a perennial herb that has a yellow flower. It is very popular and instantly recognizable. Torn leaves and flowers ooze out white latex.

Habitat

Hardy weed that is found almost everywhere around the world.

Edible

They are often used as a salad green for its distinct taste and nutrient-rich composition. Dandelion leaf/roots tea has multiple benefits. Leaves can also be used to make stir-fries.

Harvest

Leaves, roots, and flowers can be harvested upon maturation.

Uses

The root decoction can be used as a blood purifier and as a liver tonic. It can be used to treat inflammation and congestion. It can also be used to treat urinary tract infections, gallbladder problems, appetite loss, etc. Root extract can bring down cholesterol. Has good diuretic properties and can perform better (or equal) to prescription drugs.

Horse Nettle

Solanaceae (Solanum carolinense L.)

Identification

It grows up to 24" and produces a tiny yellow fruit. The leaves have spines and are rough. According to traditional medicines, leaves that have spines should never be consumed as they are generally toxic (in this case, they are).

Habitat

Horse nettle is commonly found in open fields, cultivated fields, well-drained area, and even in cultivated area to attract

Harvest

The leaves can be crushed to and used as an insect repellant. The wilted plants have been used by Cherokee topically on poison ivy.

Wild Carrot

Umbelliferaceae (Daucus Carota L.)

Identification

It is a biennial with featherlike and deeply cut leaves. The root and torn leaves generally smell like carrots. In the second year, the plant bears white flowers that smell like carrots. It is also known as Queen Anne's lace.

Habitat

Found in vacant lots, meadows, roadsides, etc.

Edible

The florets can be added to salads to get bioflavonoids, the seeds can also be added to salads and juices and the root is woody but edible. It is a great survival food if nothing else is available.

Caution

Many poisonous plants look like Daucus Carota. This plant also looks like hemlock, do not harvest unless you are perfectly sure.

Uses

The extracts can be used as an anti-wrinkle agent. The plant can be infused and used to wash sores, wounds, and even hair. Some people use leaves to purge bowels. The leaves also contain carotenoids that can prevent cancer. Tea made with whole plant and seeds can be used to treat stones, cystitis, and other urinary problems. Seeds can also be used as an anti-flatulent. The oil of the seeds is used in many cosmetics and skin products. The un-juiced carrots can be used as an antidiabetic.

Goldenrod

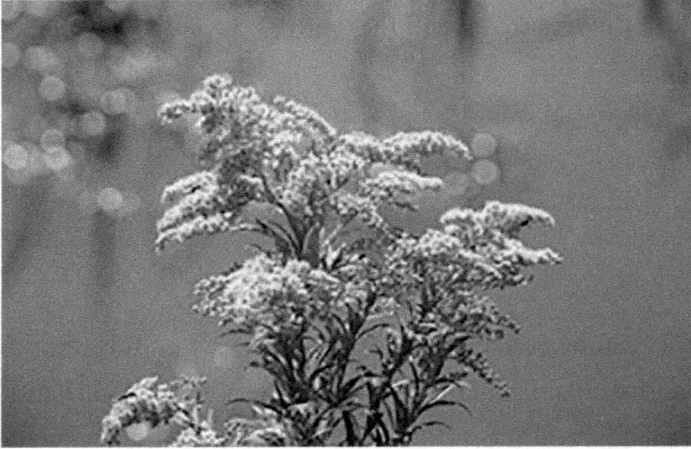

Asteraceae (Solidago Canadensis L.; Solidago spp.)

Identification

There is a multitude of species, and almost all are perennial. The leaves are sharp-toothed and are lance-shaped with three veins. The flowers grow in triangular bunches. The flowers bloom from July to September.

Habitat

It is found in vacant lots, meadows, fields, railroads, edges of fields, etc.

Edible

The shoots, leaves, and seeds are edible. The flowers can be used to make teas or can be used to make tea or can be added to salads and other dishes.

Uses

Goldenrod should not be confused with ragweed. The tea made with its leaves and flowers can be used against allergies. The dried flowers and leaves can also be applied to wounds. The flowers and leaves can be used for UTIs and kidney stones. The plant also has anti-inflammatory properties.

Caution

The plant rarely can lead to allergic reactions. People with kidney and bladder problems should not use it. Always consult a doctor before using the plant.

Stinging Nettle

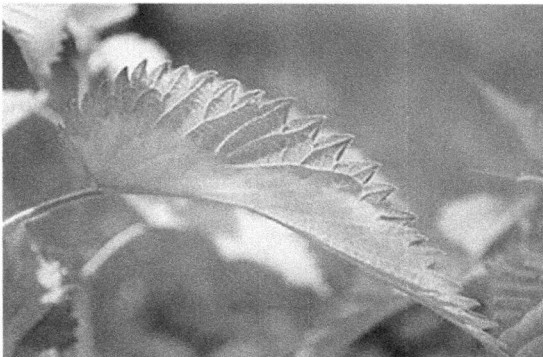

Urticaceae (Urtica dioica L.)

Identification

Another perennial that grows up to 5' tall. It is covered with stinging hair and has a heart (or oval) shaped leaves of dark green color. It has a lot of seeds.

Edible

The young shoots in spring and fall can be cooked and consumed. The hardened nettles can be used in soup base etc. While making soup with hardened material, discard it after 20-25 minutes.

Harvest

Harvest the young shoots in fall or spring.

Uses

Nettles are full of minerals and can be used to treat allergies. The infusion has expectorant qualities and can be used to cure cough and asthma. The dried parts can be used to clean wounds. Eating nettles may be useful for the health of the hair. In traditional Russian medicine, it is used to treat hepatitis. The root can be used to reduce the size of kidney stones. The decoction of the seeds can be used to prevent urination in children (involuntary).

Traditionally nettle has been used to thrash arthritic joints as it causes pain and reduces inflammation. It can bring temporary relief, but it is not recommended.

Caution

It can cause irritation and allergies in some people.

Strawberry

Rosaceae (Fragaria virginiana, F. vesca, Californica)

Identification

They have small, white flowers with five petals and five sepals. The sepals are pointed, triangular, and hairy. The leaves are present in sets of three and are hairy too. The fruit becomes red when ripe and edible.

Habitat

Strawberries can be found in the wild in meadows, open woods, etc.

Harvest

The fruits can be harvest around early June. The best time to harvest is in the spring, as it will provide you with a robust harvest.

Edible

Strawberries are edible and are full of fiber and vitamin C. It is a healthy option for people who are trying to lose weight or who are trying to control their blood sugar levels. It can be used in a variety of ways, including smoothies, pancakes, etc. It can be eaten raw as well.

Uses

Traditionally strawberry has been used by Native Americans to treat kidney infection, gout, and scurvy. The roots were used to treat malaria. In many parts of the world, the leaves are used to make tea, which has anti-diarrhea properties.

Strawberries contain a lot of antioxidants and can lower cholesterol.

Yarrow

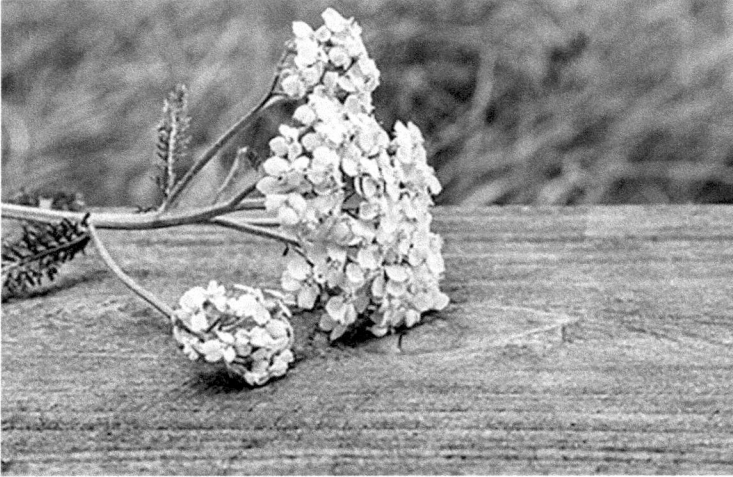

Asteraceae (Achillea millefolium L.)

Identification

It is a perennial with soft leaves and grows about 4' in height. The flowers are white and grow in a cluster. They are fragrant and have five petals.

Habitat

It is easily found around streams, woods, mountain slopes, and montane areas.

Edible

It is technically edible but rarely consumed. It is often used to flavor various liquors and is considered to be a secret ingredient. Tea made with yarrow can save you from a lot of infections.

Harvest

The aerial parts can be harvested once the flowering begins.

Uses

Native Americans consider yarrow as the most important herb and use almost all parts of it. Native

American Uses

Yarrow is ranked as one of the most important herbs used by Native Americans. An infusion of the aerial parts of the plant can be used to treat various infections, including fever, colds, flu, and also serves as a great diuretic. The infusion can also be used to wash wounds, bites, and stings. A root decoction is used to clean pimples. Tea made from leaves can be used to induce sleep and to stop diarrhea. Dry, as well as fresh leaves, can be used as a poultice for wounds. Leaf infusion can be used as a shampoo.

The tea made from flowers and leaves can increase perspiration and can bring down inflammation internally and externally. Chinese people use tea to safeguard themselves from thrombosis. In modern medicine, the leaves can be used to treat problems related to liver, appetite, and dyspepsia. In many parts of the world, the plant is used as a tonic, antispasmodic, digestive aid, and cleaning wounds. The aerial parts have carminative properties.

Caution

Do not use if pregnant or lactating. The tea can often lead to photosensitivity, which means being too sensitive to light. The tea sometimes also contains thujone, a liver toxin that is also a carcinogen. Check for allergies before using them.

Burdock

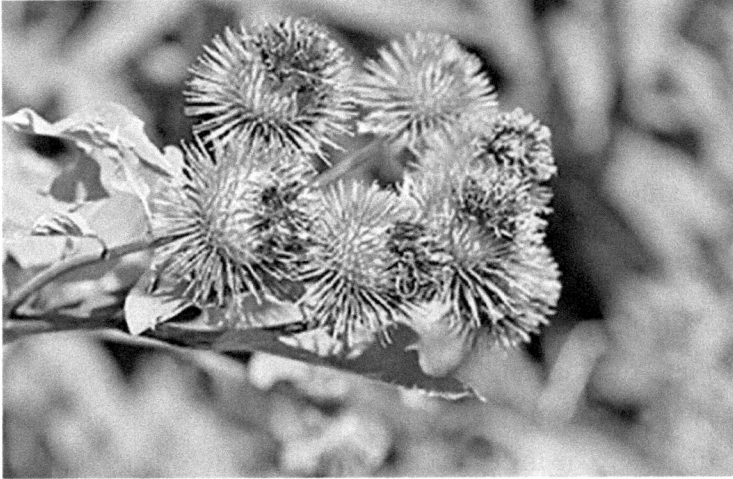

Asteraceae (Arctium lappa L.)

Identification

It is a biennial plant that produces heart-shaped leaves in the first year that grow directly from the taproot. In the second year, the growth increases with multiple branches. Flowers are red with inward bracts that produce seed capsules commonly known as burrs. These have spines that get attached to trousers, animal fur, etc. To plant the seeds, the burrs must be broken.

Habitat

It is generally found in the temperate zones and northern hemisphere. It is also found alongside roads, gardens, and almost everywhere.

Edible

The roots are edible. They are generally twenty inches or longer. Slice the roots diagonally and cook them (steam/fry) for a delicious and nutrient-rich side-dish.

Harvesting

The roots can be harvested in spring or autumn in the first year.

Uses

Burdock can be used to treat various skin conditions and immunity-related problems. Root oil and leaf infusion both work great for skin problems. It also acts as a detoxifier and can strengthen the lymphatic system, stomach, liver, etc. According to some studies, it also has anti-cancer properties.

Caution

Do not use if you are pregnant or lactating. The roots can be difficult to digest.

Chicory

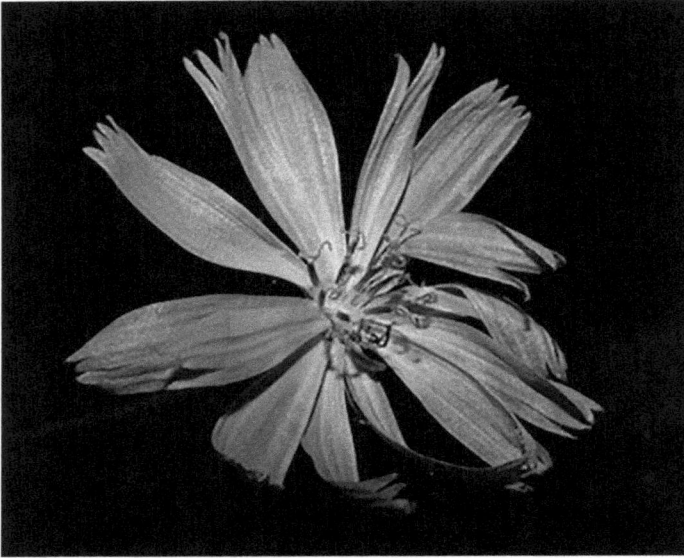

Asteraceae (Cichorium intybus L.)

Identification

It is generally a perennial but can be biennial as well. The leaves are shaped like a lance. Flowers are blue but, in rare cases, can be pink or white. It has a taproot akin to the roots of dandelion.

Habitat

Waste grounds, fields, and meadows.

Harvest

The roots and flowers can be harvested once the plant is in the second year.

Edible

The flowers are a bit bitter and can be added to teas, salads, etc. The root is used to make dry Cajun coffee. Flowers can be sprinkled over meat dishes as a garnish.

Uses

The dried/fresh root is used as a dietetic, diuretic, and laxative. The root tea improves digestion. It can also be used to treat headaches. In Homeopathy, the roots are used to reduce blood sugar and for liver and gallbladder problems. It has anti-inflammatory properties. Can lower cholesterol, although more studies are needed.

Dock

Polygonaceae (Rumex crispus L.)

Identification

Yellow dock (0r curly dock) has long, large, wavy, lance-shaped leaves that have a distinctly sour taste. The followers are present on green seed heads and bloom profusely from May to September. The root is deep, large, and pale yellow.

Habitat

It can be found in vacant lots, yards, roadsides, etc.

Harvest

Young leaves should be harvested as soon as possible as they get bitter with age. Seeds can be ground together to make mush.

Uses

It was often used as a treatment for arthritis. Cherokees used the roots for diarrhea. Cooked seeds, too, can be used to treat diarrhea. It is a good blood purifier. Naturopaths recommend roots to pregnant women as a source of iron.

The leaves and roots can stimulate digestion. It can be used against multiple skin problems. It is often combined with dandelion roots to make homemade cosmetics. It stimulates liver activity.

Caution

Do not consume too many dock leaves as they contain high amounts of tannin. They can prove to be bad for the kidneys and other body organs if eaten in excess.

Lemon Balm

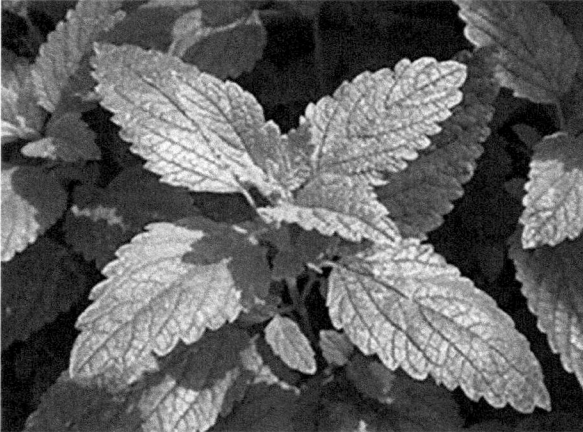

Lamiaceae (Melissa officinalis L.)

Identification

A small perennial, it has small two-petalled flowers that smell of lemon. The leaves, too, have a citrus-like smell. The seeds are brown while the stem is square and erect. Leaves are generally oval and abundant and it blooms profusely in summers.

Habitat

It is a garden plant that thrives almost everywhere. It can be found all over North America.

Edible

Leaf buds, flowers, etc. can be added to a variety of recipes and can be eaten raw. Mature leaves are used to make tea, baths, etc.

Harvest

The leaves, shoots, and flowers can be harvested around the time of blooming.

Uses

It contains a lot of phytochemicals that can soothe and relax muscles and is often used as a calming agent. It can reduce stress and blood pressure (unproven). It is often used to treat insomnia and agitation. It can also be used as an antiviral drug. However, not to be used when pregnant or lactating, as it is considered a uterine stimulant.

Caution

It can inhibit the functioning of the thyroid gland. It is not recommended for pregnant or lactating women.

Common Milkweed

Asclepiadaceous (Asclepias syriaca L.)

Identification

It is a medium-sized perennial with many different species. Flowers are pink and bloom in clusters. The flowers and seedpods both look striking.

Habitat

It is commonly found in waste grounds, railroads, roadsides, cornfields, deserts, dunes, gardens, etc.

Harvest

Shoots, flowers, and leaves can be used once the plant starts to bloom. The seedpods can be harvest upon maturation.

Edible

Flower buds can be harvested before they open and cooked like cabbage. The seedpods can be cooked after boiling. It is recommended to wash the pods thrice with boiling water. The flowers can be stored and used in winter in stews. In homeopathy, it can be used to treat dropsy, edema, etc. In Chinese medicine, it is used to treat bronchitis, tonsillitis, urethritis, pneumonia, and is used as an anti-septic.

Uses

The dried roots can be used to reduce palpitations (but should only be used under medical supervision).

Caution

Certain species can be toxic. Do not consume without consulting a botanist. The root decoction of certain species can lead to allergies.

Catnip

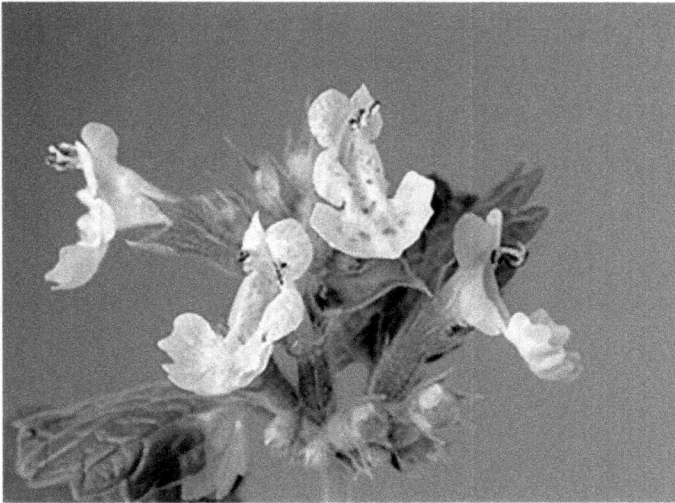

Lamiaceae (Nepeta cataria L.)

Identification

It is a perennial plant that can grow up to 3.5'. It is generally erect and has many stems. The leaves are greenish-grey, which makes it look a bit like sage. Flowers are present in a large cluster.

Habitat

It can be found along roadsides, waste ground, gardens, yards, etc.

Harvest

The leaves can be harvested when young.

Edible

Leaves can be used to make tea.

Uses

The aerial parts are used to make a bitter but antispasmodic infusion. The tea made with leaves and flowers has a slight sedative effect and the infusion also has anti-flatulent properties. It can reduce menstrual cramps. It is often used to treat upset stomach and colic in children. It can be converted into a tincture and used to reduce arthritic pain. The tea is also good for the urinary system and stimulates the gallbladder. It is often combined with elderflowers to treat infections. It can be combined with hops and valerian roots and used as a sleeping aid and as a relaxant.

Caution

Avoid if you are pregnant or a lactating mother.

Notes

If you plan to plant catnip in your garden, grow it indoors first and let it become at least a foot tall. If you plant it directly, cats will attack it.

Chamomile

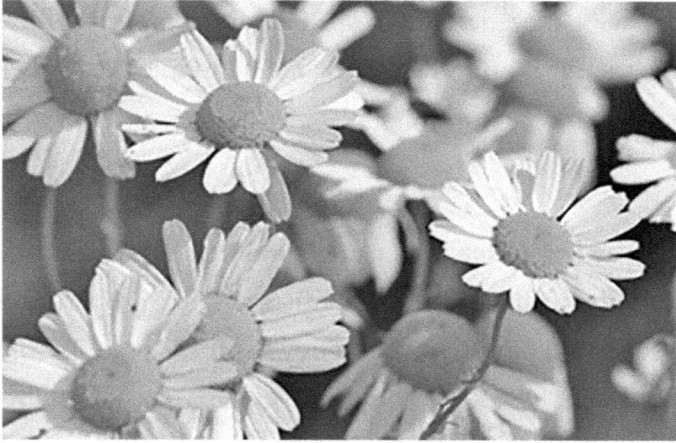

Asteraceae (Matricaria matricarioides; Chamomilla recutita L.; Chamaemelum nobile L.)

Identification

Wild chamomile is also known as pineapple weed. It has small yellow flowers and does not have the white rays present in regular chamomile. The rayless flowers smell of pineapple and the leaves are spread low.

Habitat

Is easily found around pathways, roadsides, waste grounds, and similar places. It can also be found in mountainous areas.

Harvest

The flowers and leaves should be harvested when fresh and young. The leaves get bitter with age.

Edible

The herb can be used both fresh and dry, but fresh flowers are preferred. It is far more effective than chamomile. It can be used in soups too.

Uses

Pineapple weed is quite similar to chamomile and is used as it. The tea made with fresh flowers has antispasmodic properties and can prevent ulcers, aid digestion, and relieve arthritis pain. Warm tea can also be used to reduce toothache. Native Americans used the herb to relieve stomach aches. The infusion made with flowers and leaves can reduce menstrual cramps. The infusion is also used to treat eczema, abrasions, acne, and inflammations. It is used to prepare ointments and lotions to treat wounds, sore gums, sore nipples, and other forms of inflammations. Many people used it topically to treat hemorrhoids.

Caution

This herb is often used as an antiallergic herb, but in some cases, it may lead to allergies. In fact, it can even lead to anaphylactic shock in some people. If you are allergic to ragweed, stay away from this plant.

Echinacea

Asteraceae (Echinacea purpurea L. Moench; E. angustafolia DC)

Identification

It is medium length perennial that produces beautiful purple flowers. The bracts look like thorn tips. The leaves can be opposite or alternate and generally have smooth margins. The root is a rhizome that has a yellowish center which is covered with a bark-like skin. The plant is also known as purple coneflower.

Habitat

Is generally found in central and eastern states in the wild. It is cultivated as a garden plant throughout the nation.

Harvest

The roots and flowers can be harvested once the flowers are in bloom.

Uses

The roots were used to treat snakebites. The boiled root water is often used as a treatment for sore throats. Mashed roots can be used to treat infections. Root infusion was once upon a time used to treat gonorrhea. Leaves, roots, and flowers are used commercially to make preparations that are used to treat flu, colds, bronchitis, coughs, fever, UTIs, wounds, burns, etc. The plant has anti-inflammatory properties. It can boost immunity if used regularly.

It can be used internally to treat fungal infections and various skin diseases. It can also be used to treat boils, slow-healing wounds, gangrene, and sinusitis. It can be applied topically for acne.

Caution

Do not use if pregnant or lactating. It can lead to fetal malformation and abortion. Always consult your physician before beginning any new herb and do not use if you have an active autoimmune disease. Do not use if you are allergic to daisy or aster family.

Evening Primrose

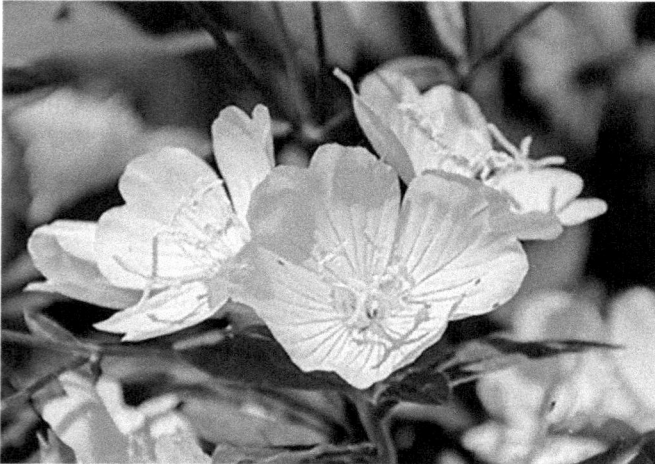

Onagraceae (Oenothera biennis L.)

Identification

This is a biennial plant that has turnip-like fleshy roots. In the first year, the plant does not flower and is just a rosette of leaves. In the second year, the plant grows erect and produces large capsules full of seeds in autumn. It has lance-shaped oblong leaves that are finely dentate. The flowers are fragrant and yellow and they bloom in the evening. Fruits are oblong and contain sharp black seeds.

Habitat

It can be found in the prairies, gardens, waste grounds, roadsides, etc.

Harvest

The root shoot is harvest in the first year for the best results. The leaves can be harvested whenever they are tender and new.

Edible

The leaves, fruit, and roots all are edible. The root tastes best when harvested young. The tender leaves can be added to salads, while the older leaves are tough and should be cooked before consuming. Immature seeds capsules can be cooked like okra.

Uses

The warm root poultice was used by the Native Americans to treat piles. The seed oil can be used to lower cholesterol and it is said to clear arterial obstructions too. It is often used to treat psoriasis and eczema. The oil is demulcent and anticoagulant.

Evening primrose oil is often used by women suffering from recurring breast cysts. It can also reduce insulin dependency in children. The oil is good for the liver and can improve its function, especially in the case of alcoholics. Vaginal suppositories made of this oil are used to relax and soften the cervix before childbirth.

Caution

Large doses may lead to diarrhea, headaches, nausea, indigestion, etc. Do not use it if you have schizophrenia or use epileptogenic drugs. There have been no long-term studies regarding the effects of evening primrose oil on pregnant and lactating people, so it is better to avoid.

Motherwort

Lamiaceae (Leonurus cardiaca L.)

Identification

It is a straight growing perennial that belongs to the mint family. The stem is squarish, hollow, and hairy while the leaves are lobed and toothed. The leaves are dark green on the top and light green underneath. The plant produces small red flowers from April to August. Leaves, if crushed, give out a strange odor.

Habitat

Originally from Europe, it has now spread throughout the nation and is often found on the edges of the lawn, waste ground, roadsides, etc.

Harvest

Leaves, stem, and flowers should be collected when the plant starts to bloom.

Edible

It is technically edible, although rarely eaten. Certain users consume the seeds as they contain fatty acids and beta-carotene. Pregnant and lactating women should avoid consuming the seeds because they are stimulating.

Uses

They are used in traditional Chinese medicine to tone the muscles of the heart. It can also be used to treat urinary cramps, dysmenorrhea, amenorrhea, and common weakness. The ancient Greeks used this herb to treat anxiety and stress in pregnant women, but modern medicine warns against this practice as the herb has uterus-stimulating effects.

It has antibacterial and antifungal properties and is used to get rid of both internal and external organisms. The aerial parts can be infused to treat heart palpitations and asthma. It is also used by people who suffer from thyroid dysfunction. It is antispasmodic, hypotensive, laxative, diuretic, sedative, and an emmenagogue.

Caution

As stated earlier, pregnant and lactating women should not use it as it can stimulate the uterus.

Foxglove

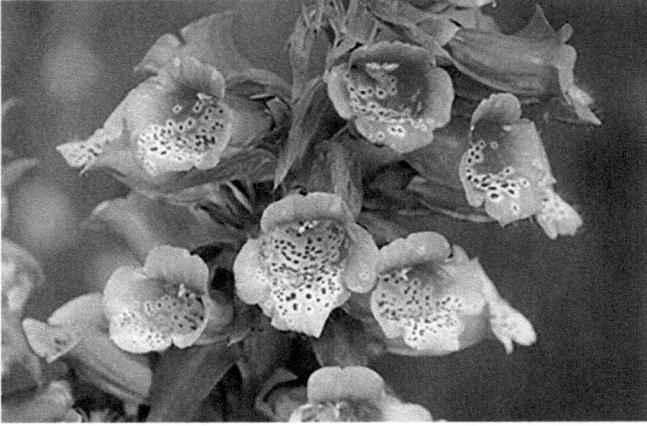

Plantaginaceae (Digitalis purpurea L.)

Identification

It is a biennial plant with hairy lance-shaped leaves that grow in clusters in the wild. When the plant is not flowering, the leaves appear like comfrey, dock, or mullein leaves, however, beware, the leaves of digitalis are toxic. Flowers are elegant and are often purple to white. Their glove-like appearance is reflected in their name. They typically flower in their second year.

Habitat

It is one of the most recognized mountain flowers that grow along roadsides. It is also an ornamental plant and is frequently found in gardens.

Harvest

Young leaves can be harvested throughout the growing period.

Not edible.

Uses

The Celtics used the powder made with leaves as a cardiac glycoside. Overdose can cause vomiting, nausea, fainting, slow pulse, and in some cases, even death. It is used topically to treat ulcers, wounds, headaches, tumors, abscesses, etc. The plant has also been used as a lethal poison. In modern medicine, this plant and its medical properties are considered to be obsolete.

Caution

The plant is toxic for animals too. The flowers are so toxic that even the water in the vase of cut flowers becomes a potent poison.

Pokeweed

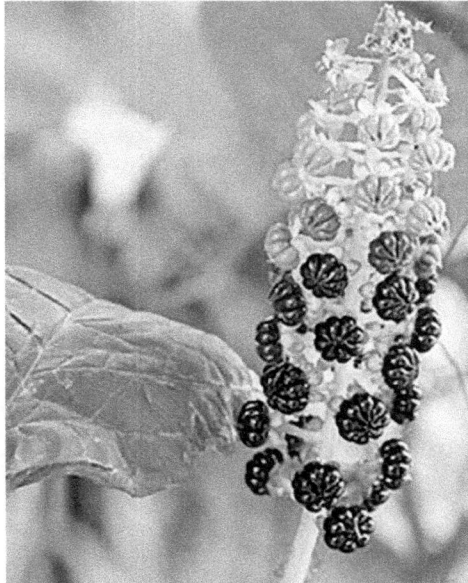

Phytolaccaceae (Phytolacca americana L.)

Identification

It a large perennial with a smooth, thick, and reddish stem that grows up to 10' tall. The stems have grooves and are hollow. The root is thick and long while the leaves are lance-shaped and can be ovate. When crushed, the leaves produce a musty smell. The flowers have a calyx but do not have corolla. They are greenish-white. The berries are borne in a cluster and turn black (or purple) upon maturation.

Habitat

It can be found on roadsides, waste grounds, gardens, and fields.

Harvest

The leaves should be harvested before the petioles, and stem start to turn purple. Berries, seeds, and roots are toxic and should not be consumed.

Edible

Boil the young shoot twice before consuming. The amount of lectin increases with the maturation of the plant. Cooking and digestive juices can destroy almost all of the lectin, yet caution is a must. It is delicious green that can also be found commercially. Tender and young stems can be pickled and blanched. The leaves are rich in minerals and Vitamin C. In fact, they contain three times more Vitamin C than a lemon. The Cherokee used to make a drink using the ripe berries, powdered cornmeal, and sour grapes.

Uses

Natives used the roots as a poultice over rheumatoid joints. Infusion of roots is used to treat ulcerated wounds, eczema, and to bring down swelling. The plant has emetic and laxative properties. The parts of the plant are used as antiarthritic and purgative. The leaves are currently being researched as a possible treatment of viral infections and cancer. Homeopathic doses are available for inflammations, rheumatism, fever, and certain infections. The saponins of roots are emetic. The root extract can be used as an immunity booster.

Caution

Overdose can lead to respiratory problems, diarrhea, dizziness, hypotension, tachycardia, thirst, spasm, vomiting, and in particular, high doses- death. Berries are extremely toxic to children, and just one berry can make a child severely ill. More than ten berries can prove to be fatal. Yet the berries are used by the food industry as a colorant.

Amaranth, Red Root

Amaranthaceae (Amaranthus retroflexus L.)

Identification

It is a tall plant that looks a bit like certain weeds. It has grayish, alternate leaves, and the flowers grow in hairy bracts. The size of the leaves decreases towards the top of the plant. Seeds are numerous and tiny, black colored and the lower stem and taproot are reddish. The leaves are rough to touch.

Habitat

Is widely cultivated in South America and Mexico. Many different species grow across the margin of fields, prairies, etc.

Harvest

The leaves and young shoots should be harvested when fresh. The seeds can be harvested carefully upon maturation. The seeds are very tiny and should be harvested with proper tools.

Edible

The leaves and shoots can be eaten raw or can be cooked. They can also be dried and eaten in winter. The seeds can be incorporated into flour and cereal. Seeds can also be used in muffins, bread, and other baked products. Black, mature seeds are used to make pinole with water and cornmeal.

Uses

It is considered to be a sacred plant by Native Indians and is consumed ritualistically in combination with green corn in a variety of ceremonies. The leaves are used to treat excessive menstruation. The herb is an astringent and can prove to be beneficial in ulcers, diarrhea, and inflammations of the throat and mouth. In modern medicine, it has little to no proven uses, but it has no health hazards either can be consumed freely.

Notes

The plant grows well in gardens and propagates thanks to the high number of seeds easily. The seeds should be added to salads, baked goods, stir-fries, etc.

Passion Flower

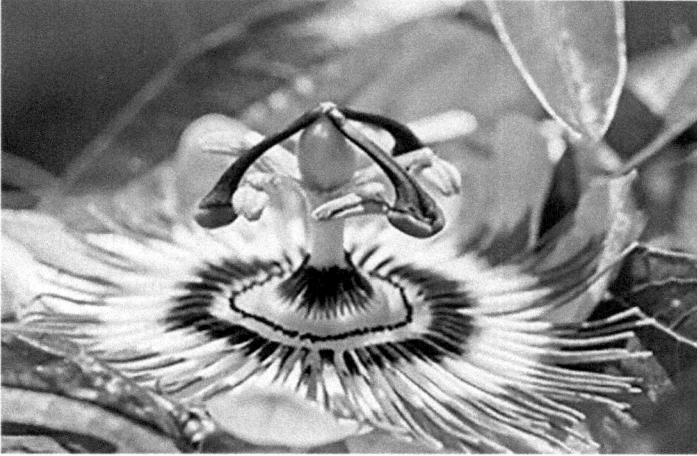

Passifloraceae (Passiflora incarnata L.)

Identification

Dozens of varieties differ on minor grounds. It is a woody, perennial vine. The bark is striated and longitudinal. Leaves have petioles, are serrated, and grow alternate. The underside of the leaf is hairier than the top. The leaf blades have bumps, which are also known as floral nectaries. Flowers are striking with multiple spokes, shaped like a wheel.

Habitat

It is often found in forests and other places throughout the world. Most of the species are subtropical or tropical but can thrive in temperate zones too. Numerous species are found throughout the world. It is found in the wild in the southeast zone of the United States.

Harvest

The leaves can be harvested anytime but the flowers should be harvested fresh. The fruit can be harvested upon maturation.

Edible

The tea made using flowers and leaves has slight sedative properties. The fruit can be eaten fresh, raw, or can be made into a juice. Mexicans mix the fruit with flour or cornmeal to make gruel. Leaves are consumed by Native Americans and are generally boiled and then sautéed.

Uses

The infusion made with dried or fresh aerial parts of the herb has sedative properties. It can be used to treat insomnia and nervousness. It has an antispasmodic effect, which makes it good for the digestive system. The crushed root is often used to treat earache. The crushed root can also be used to apply as a poultice on boils, contusions, and cuts. The whole plant, combined with Epsom salts, can be used as sedative baths. The tea made with aerial parts, and roots can be used to treat hemorrhoids. In animal studies, it was found that it can inhibit the motility of organisms and has antispasmodic and sedative properties. It is now used to treat insomnia and nervousness. It can be used to treat 'hysteria.'

Purslane

Portulacaceae (Portulaca oleracea L.)

Identification

A creeping succulent that spreads on the ground. Stems have multiple branches and are often reddish. The leaves are thick, long, smooth, fleshy, teardrop-shaped, and shiny. There are multiple varieties, but the most common one has yellowish flowers. The blooms are seen throughout June to November.

Harvest

The parts of the plant can be harvested anytime, although fresh harvesting is ideally recommended.

Habitat

This plant is seen all over the nation, often on waste grounds and in gardens. It can be plucked and eaten right off the ground.

Edible

It is a common garden plant. It is a great addition to salads, soups, etc. Contains high quantities of omega-3 acids. The leaves can be consumed raw or can be eaten as a cooked vegetable. It is often added to meat recipes and stews. It can also be boiled to make soup. It can be dried and then reconstituted to be used a winter food.

Uses

It can be used as a skin lotion and poultice. The decoction made with the whole plant can be used to treat worms. The juice of the whole plant can be used as a tonic and can be used to treat earaches. The infusion made with the stems and leaves can be used to stop diarrhea. The plant can be crushed and applied to bruises and burns as a poultice. The Decoction of the complete plant can be used as an antiseptic wash. Purslane can be used to treat stomachache. The plant contains many different essential fatty acids, which can help you prevent inflammatory diseases and disorders such as diabetes, heart disease, and arthritis. The extract from this plant is often used in cosmetics.

Saint-John's-Wort

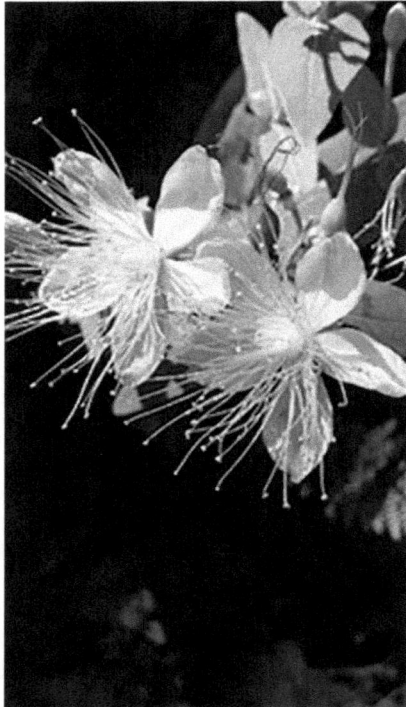

Hyperacaceae (Hypericum perforatum L.)

Identification

It has a woody stem that is stiff, erect, and reddish. The leaves are attached at the base and are ovate and covered with glands. These glands can be seen if the leaves are held towards the sun. The glands look like tiny perforations. The stems bear clusters of yellow flowers with five sepals each and blossoms have multiple stamens. The seeds are cylindrical, brown or black, and are covered with markings.

Habitat

This plant can be found almost everywhere. It is commonly observed near riverbanks, stream banks, waste grounds, roadsides, etc. many varieties are grown in gardens as well.

Harvest

Harvest early. The flowers should be harvest fresh and can be dried later in the shade.

Uses

The decoction made with the whole plant was used to induce abortion. It may contain antibacterial, antiviral, and other similar properties. It was considered to be an astringent, anti-inflammatory, and antidiarrheal. Has been used in Greece traditionally to drive away spirits. The infusion made with flowers can treat insomnia and can dispel lethargy. It can also calm nerves and relieves stress. The tea was used to treat anxiety, sciatica, shingles, anxiety, and fibrositis in the past. The crushed flowers and leaves were stuffed in the nose to stop nosebleeds.

In modern medicines, several studies have been made across Europe that show that the plant can be used to treat mild depression. The drug can also be used for weight loss, fatigue, anxiety, menopausal symptoms, and to improve sleep.

An infusion made with leaves and flowers can be used externally for its wound-healing and cooling properties. It is good for burns, infections, sprains, bruises, neuralgia, cramps, tendonitis, etc. Studies have shown that it is effective against various microbes such as herpes simplex I and II, influenza, poliovirus, retrovirus, murine cytomegalovirus, sindbis virus, gram-negative and gram-positive bacteria, and hepatitis C. Exposure to ultraviolet light can enhance antimicrobial activity.

Note: It is available over-the-counter as a dietary supplement. It is recommended to consult a health practitioner to find out the proper dosage and usage.

Caution

Should not be used to treat bipolar or severe depression. It can have certain side-effects such as restlessness, gastrointestinal irritation, allergy, etc. The supplement may reduce the activity of certain drugs such as oral contraceptives, non-sedating antihistamines, antiepileptic, antiretroviral, calcium channel blockers, chemotherapeutics, cyclosporine, certain antifungals, and antibiotics. Long-term abuse of St. John's wort can lead to various negative consequences on health. Do not use it without proper consultation.

Heal-All

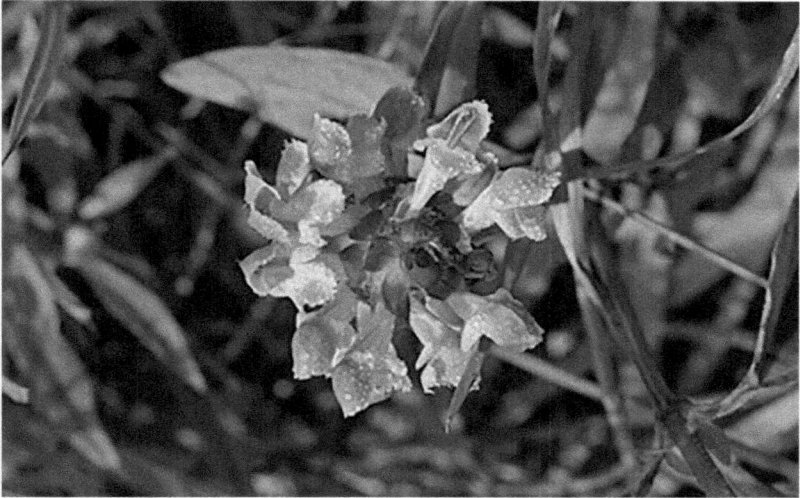

Lamiaceae (Prunella vulgaris L.)

Identification

It is perennial with a squarish stem that may fall and creep once mature. Leaves are toothed and lance-shaped while the flowers can range from blue to violet. The plant is also known as self-heal.

Habitat

It is found throughout the nation in lawns, waste ground, fields, wetlands, woods, etc.

Harvest

Harvest the shoots and flowers when fresh.

Edible

The infusion made with the aerial parts of the plant was used as a beverage by the Thompson First People. The flowers and leaves can be added to salads and juices.

Uses

The Chinese have been using this herb since ancient times for liver problems and to improve the health and function of the liver in general. The infusion made with the whole plant can stimulate gallbladder and liver and can promote healing. Heal-all is used by many practitioners to treat excessive menstruation. It is also used externally by people to treat cuts, burns, sore throats, and sores. The infusion made with the whole plant can be used as a gargle to treat ulcers of the throat and the mouth.

The dried aerial parts can be used to make tea to treat diarrhea. The extracts of this herb can be used to treat gingivitis.

Spiderwort

Commelinaceae (Tradescantia ohioensis L.; T. occidentalis [Britt.], Smyth; T. pinetorum Greene)

Identification

It is a perennial plant with no stem. The leaves are numerous, long, and sword-like and grow from the base and the flowers are deep blue, orchid-like. They open in the morning and begin to shut by afternoon.

There are four species found in North America. The plant is also known as a spider plant or widow's tears.

Habitat

Various species are found throughout the nation. T. occidentalis is generally found in the central states, while Trandescantia virginiana is found along roadsides, railroads, prairies, fields, etc.

Harvest

The shoots should be harvested when tender. The flowers can be harvested throughout the year, but it is recommended to harvest them in the morning. Harvest the root once the plant starts to bloom.

Edible

The tender shoots can be cooked or eaten raw. The flowers can be added to salads or can be made into stir-fries and they can also be eaten raw. There are many other ways of cooking the flowers, including fritters, juices, etc.

Uses

The tea made using the roots mentioned above can be used to treat female kidney disorders and various other stomach problems. It is also used as a laxative. The infusion made with aerial parts is used to treat stomachache. The aerial plants were crushed and used as a poultice over stings and insect bites in ancient times. The infusion of this plant is supposed to be an aphrodisiac.

Uses

The flowers have flavonoids which contain health-enhancing and protecting properties. It is a good diuretic and can lower blood pressure and improve overall circulation too. The young shoots are mucilaginous, which can help to treat sore throat and sinus problems. It is used in traditional Chines Medicine to treat swelling.

Wild Yam

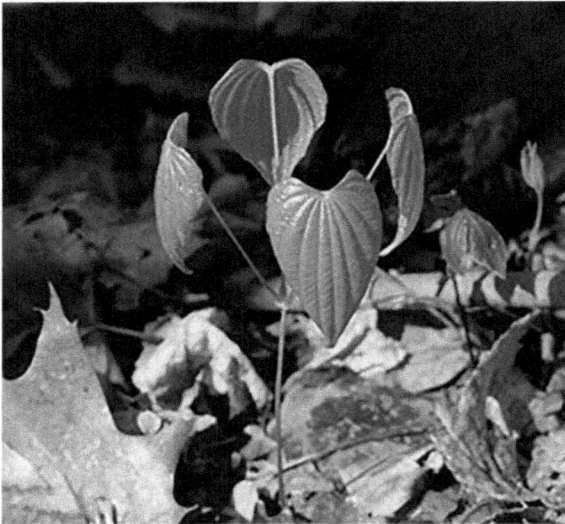

Dioscoreaceae (Dioscorea villosa L.; D. composita Hemsl)

Identification

It is large, sprawling, a perennial vine with a reddish-brown stem. The leaves are heart-shaped and alternate and they are hairy underneath, while the top is smooth. The greenish-yellow flowers are small and gendered. The root is cylindrical and has multiple uses.

Habitat

Wild Yam is found throughout the continent of North America. It has multiple species that grow from Canada to the southern United States in tropical, subtropical, and temperate weather.

Harvest

Dig out the root once the flowers start to bloom.

Edible

Wild yams are often a part of Chinese medicinal soups. They are bitter and can be toxic.

Uses

The decoction made with the root was used as an analgesic for postpartum pain and during delivery by Meskwakis Indians. In ancient Chinese medicine, the dried root slices are used with polygonatum to treat dysmenorrhea. The root is also used to treat pain associated with menstruation by the indigenous people of South America. The decoction can also be used as a digestive aid, for muscle cramping, and for arthritis. It is supposed to have warming, antispasmodic, anti-inflammatory, antiarthritic, and diuretic properties. It contains a chemical called diosgenin, which forms the material for the birth control pill. Naturopaths prescribe the tea for IBS. The root decoction is used by practitioners to treat nocturnal emissions, chronic fatigue, neurasthenia, neurosis, insomnia, and feelings of inadequacy. The smashed roots can be used as a poultice for boils, abscesses, and skin sores.

Caution

Do not consume if you are pregnant or lactating. Similarly, do not consume if you suffer from constipation or have blood pressure problems. Consult with a health practitioner before using wild yam internally.

Baptisia

Fabaceae (Baptisia australis L. R. Br. ex Ait. f.; B. tinctorial L.)

Identification

It is a shrub-like, albeit tall perennial that grows up to 5' in height. The leaves are like a pea. It produces beautiful blue, pea-like flowers and the seedpods are indigo.

Habitat

It can be found in gardens and prairies.

Not Edible

Harvest

The roots should be harvested upon maturation.

Uses

A decoction made using the roots was used by the Natives to treat bites, wounds, and stings. It is an immune-stimulating herb which is used as a vaginal douche in traditional medicine as a treatment for vaginitis. The poultice of roots is used to treat sores caused by venereal diseases. The root infusion can be used to wash wounds but an excessive dosage can lead to vomiting and nausea. Research is going on its effects on leukocytes.

Caution

Should not be ingested as it can prove to be toxic.

California Poppy

Papaveraceae (Eschscholzia Californica Cham.)

Identification

It can be a perennial or an annual plant that can grow up to 40" tall. The leaves are scant and are bluish. They are fernlike or feathery. The flowers are solitary and are of striking shades of orange and yellow. There are hundreds of species available in the wild.

Habitat

It is found in wild on roadsides, open areas, wastelands, etc. in the area from British Columbia to California. It is grown in the garden as an ornamental plant throughout the nation.

Harvest

The aerial parts can be harvested once the flowers start to bloom.

Uses

An infusion made with the dried aerial parts of the plant can be used as a sedative. It has been traditionally to reduce nervousness, anxiety, and stress. It has diuretic and analgesic properties. Many tribes use it to treat nocturnal urination in children and certain tribes used the milky sap produced by leaves to treat toothache. The white resin produced by seedpods was rubbed on breasts to improve the production of milk. An alkaloid called Californidine derived from the plant is used as a sedative and as a sleep aid. Homeopathy practitioners use it to make preparations that are used to treat insomnia.

Caution

Do not use if pregnant or lactating.

Flax

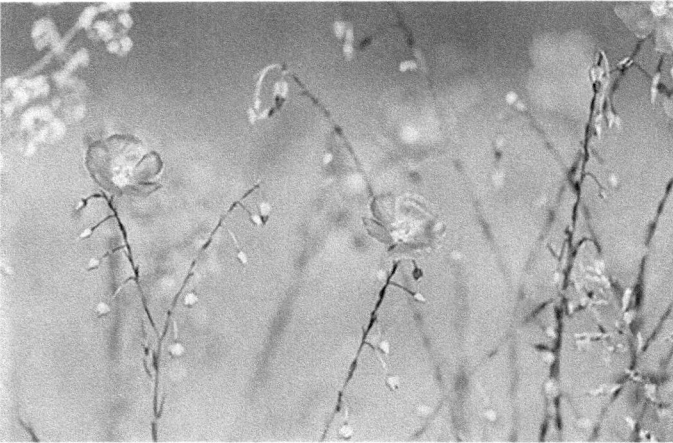

Linaceae (Linum usitatissimum L.)

Identification

It is a slender, delicate annual that has lance-shaped leaves and produces sky-blue flowers with five stamens, five petals, five sepals, and one ovary. The seeds are brown, flat, and glossy. It is also commonly known as linseed.

Habitat

It is often found in temperate zones, but it grows almost everywhere, including barns, roadsides, waste ground, etc. You can also grow these plants in your garden.

Harvest

The seeds can be harvest upon maturation.

Uses

The ancient Greeks and Romans considered flax to be a 'cure-all' medicine. Native Americans use flax as medicine and food. It was used to treat coughs, inflammation, infections, cold, urinary pain, fevers, etc. It is one of the richest plant sources of omega-3 fatty acids, narrowly topped by perilla seeds. Omega-3 boosts memory and enhances cognition. It also keeps users safe from degenerative diseases. Consuming high amounts of omega-3 and omega-6 can help you avoid inflammatory and autoimmune diseases. The husk of the seeds is used as mucilage. It contains a high amount of phenolics, which can prevent cancer, heart problems, and diabetes. It can be used to treat constipation. The oil produced from the seeds increases the levels of plasma in insulin and brings down cholesterol.

Chapter 3

Eastern Forested Areas and
Medicinal Herbs

Here is a list of some common medicinal plants that can be found in the forested areas of the United States of America. Many of these plants are transitional plants, which means they can be observed in forests as well as between the transitional zones of forests and roadsides.

Skunk Cabbage

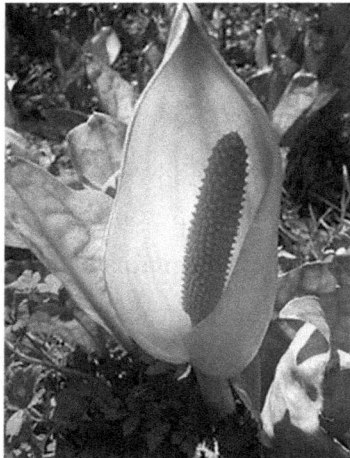

Araceae (Symplocarpus foetidus L. Nutt.)

Identification

It is a large leafy plant that has elephant-like gigantic leaves. The leaves are waxy, green, and lustrous. When torn, they smell like which gives the plant its name.

Habitat

Found majorly in wet woods, lowlands, swamps, wet coastal areas, etc. Predominantly found in Eastern states.

Harvest

The roots can be harvested after the plant blooms.

Edible

The eastern species is not used for food, but some people do consume the thoroughly dried roots. The fresh roots should not be consumed that they can cause burning sensations in the digestive tract and the mouth.

Uses

The liquid extract of the roots was once used to treat asthma and bronchitis and a tea made with dried roots is used to stop asthma, coughs, seizures, and toothache. The paste of dried roots can be used topically to stop itching. The leaves can be crushed and used as a poultice on swellings. This poultice is considered to be an antirheumatic and analgesic and the dried roots can be used to treat coughs. The stalks can be crushed to make a decoction, which can be used as a douche to improve displacement of the womb. The leaves were once upon a time chewed to treat epilepsy. The powder of dried leaves was used to treat convulsions. The liquid extract of this plant is still used to treat asthma and bronchitis. It is an expectorant, antispasmodic, diaphoretic, and sedative. Only skilled practitioners should use it as it can prove to be toxic.

Caution

It contains crystals of poisonous oxalate. The liquid from a fresh plant will lead to blistering of the skin and may burn the digestive tract severely if consumed. It can be consumed but needs extensive preparations, which ultimately does not yield a lot of food or taste. Only experts should handle this plant.

Hepatica

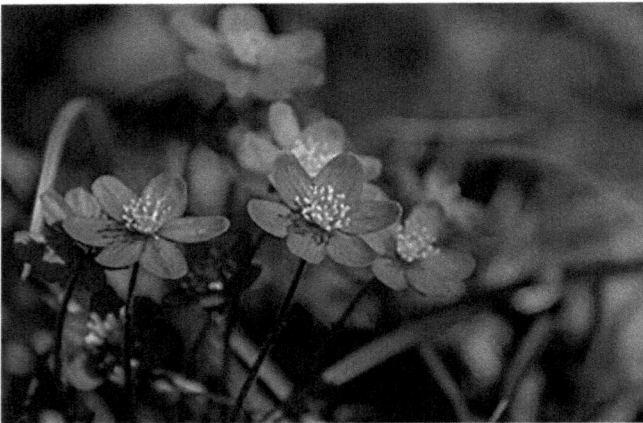

Ranunculaceae (Hepatica nobilis var. obtusa [Pursh] Steyermark, also known as H. triloba and H. americana; H. nobilis var. acuta [Pursh] Steyermark, also known as H. acutiloba)

Identification

It is a small, evergreen, perennial plant with basal leaves. The H. nobilis var. obtuse has round lobed leaves while the H. nobilis var. acuta has sharp lobed leaves. H. var. obtuse has whitish flowers while the H. var. acuta has bluish-violet flowers. This is one of the first flowers to bloom in the spring. It is also known as American liverwort.

Harvest

The leaves can be harvested fresh. Roots should be harvested upon maturation.

Habitat

It can be easily found in Eastern forests.

Uses

The Native Americans used H. nobilis var. obtusa for its laxative and emetic properties. It is also an abortifacient. It was also used as a contraceptive by the tribes. The root decoction and leaf infusions are used to treat vertigo and diarrhea. The tea made with the leaves was used to treat liver problems. It was considered to be a tonic once upon a time. The decoction was used to stimulate the uterus. It was one of the most used herbs of the 19th century. Certain modern practitioners still use it to treat gallstones and other liver problems.

Caution

The overdose of this plant is poisonous. The plant should only be used under proper medical guidance and supervision. Do not touch the plant as it may lead to dermatitis. If ingested without caution, it can cause problems to the urinary system and the intestinal tract.

Bloodroot

Papaveraceae (Sanguinaria Canadensis L.)

Identification

It is a perennial plant with thick rhizome. When cutting the rhizome gives out a red liquid. The leaves are grayish-green. The flowers bloom singly and have 8 or more white petals and it blooms in the early spring and dies out quickly.

Habitat

It is generally found in damp and rich forests.

Not Edible

Uses

The extract from this plant is warming and has antispasmodic properties. The herb was used by Native Americans to induce vomiting. The extracts of the roots were once used to treat cough, fever, rheumatism, and laryngitis. Very tiny doses were used to stimulate the appetite. It is an anesthetic. Some people used it to treat asthma, bronchitis, throat infections, and various lung problems. It contains chemical compounds known as chelerythrine and sanguinarine, which have anti-cancer properties. In research trials, it has been found that ear and nose cancers respond positively to topical applications. It is often used topically for its anti-inflammatory properties. Sanguinarine is toxic, but it has antiseptic properties and is often used in toothpaste and mouthwashes.

The exudate of the plant can be combined with water to make a thin solution. This solution, when applied topically, can repel mosquitoes for a long time.

Caution

It is toxic, which is why it is not used as an expectorant anymore.

Mayapple

Berberidaceae (Podophyllum peltatum L.)

Identification

It is an umbrella-shaped perennial with large cleft leaves. Each stalk has only two leaves with five or more lobes. The flower is white and grows under the leaf. Fruits ripe in mid or late summer and only ripe fruits are edible. It spreads profusely over the floor of forests. It is also known as American mandrake.

Habitat

Extensive ground cover in eastern forests, rich woods.

Harvest

Harvest the ripe fruit in late summers. The roots can be harvested throughout the growing season.

Edible

The fruit can be consumed in the summer when it is ripe and soft. It is difficult to find the fruit as most of the plants die before maturation. The plants that thrive do not provide a lot of yields, often producing just one fruit per plant. Many times, the fruits are harvested by forest creatures. If you do find ripe fruit, you can eat it directly. If the fruit is not ripe, cook it. The ripe fruit can be used in waffles, muffins, pies, and pancakes. It can also be used to make jellies, jams, etc.

Uses

Native Americans used tiny doses of Mayapple to treat many different illnesses. It was used to treat papillomavirus warts. It is a powerful laxative and can be used as a purgative but the root is toxic and is often used to kill worm infestations. The powder of the root is used topically on sores. In the mid-twentieth century, doctors injected resin of Mayapple in venereal warts to treat them. An antimitotic agent is present in the root extracts, which can be used to treat testicular cancer and small-cell lung cancer. P. peltatum is still used to treat genital and other warts. The leaves and roots are poisonous, and mishandling (or even regular handling) of the leaves may lead to dermatitis. P. emodi or the Himalayan Mayapple, contains high amounts of podophyllotoxin, which is a toxic drug.

Caution

Do not use without medical supervision. The drug is often absorbed through the skin and can prove to be toxic.

Wild Leeks

Liliaceae (Allium tricoccum Ait.)

Identification

This plant has blade-shaped, long leaves that grow in pairs directly from the bulb. The plant smells like onions. The leaves disappear in a few weeks and give way from the flowering stem, which produces white clusters of flowers. Around September, only black seeds remain on the top of the flowering stem. The edible bulb still stays fresh underground, though. It is also known as a ramp.

Habitat

Found profusely on the floor of Eastern forests. It is a common plant in moist forests. It can be found above seeps, in wet woods, on moist hillsides, and in similar places.

Harvest

The stems, leaves, and bulbs can be harvested upon maturation. Harvest the bulbs once the flowers are spent, and the plant has produced seeds.

Edible

The stems, leaves, and bulbs are edible and taste brilliant in soups, stews, and stir-fries. Leaves, stems, and bulbs are edible—marvelous in stews. It can also be added to martinis and pizzas. It is one of the best medicinal/edible plants, especially for the winters. It is not only filling but is healthy as well. Seeds can be harvested in the fall and you can collect them and plant them in shady corners of your garden.

The dried seeds can also be added to a pepper mill, which will add a mild flavor of garlic to your food.

Uses

The plants are used as a tonic by Native Americans. The warm juice can be used to stop earaches. The decoction of the whole plant is used to treat worms. It is also used as a tonic to treat colds. According to some sources, eating raw bulbs can help you to reduce the risk of heart disease. The chopped leaves can be added to the soup to treat the flu and cold.

Jack-in-the-Pulpit

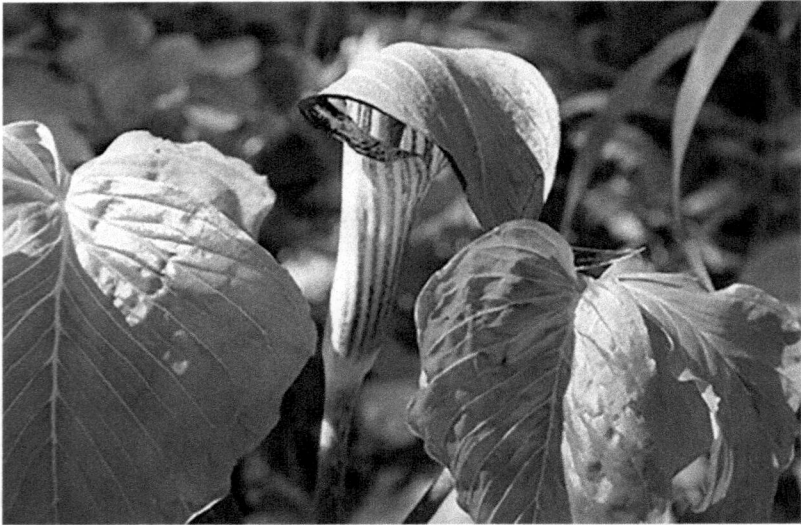

Araceae (Arisaema triphyllum L. Schott)

Identification

A small perennial with two leaves on two petioles. The leaves look like the leaves of poison ivy. Produces clusters of scarlet-colored berries.

Habitat

It can be found in rich soils and moist forests in the Eastern states of the nation.

Harvest

The roots can be harvested when tender.

Edible

The fruit of this plant is not edible and should not be consumed. The roots contain caustic calcium oxalate. Native Indians slice and dry these roots, which are said to deactivate this toxic compound. These dried slices are then cooked and consumed like potato chips.

Uses

The dried root was once upon a time used to treat various respiratory problems, including bronchitis, asthma, colds, laryngitis, and cough. The crushed root can be used to wash sores, ringworm, boils, and abscesses. A lot of varieties are still used to treat snakebite in China.

Caution

Do not consume the fresh plant ass; it contains caustic oxalates. The plant needs to be dried thoroughly before it can be consumed.

Calcium oxalate can cause burns if handled improperly.

Uva-Ursi

Ericaceae (Arctostaphylos uva-ursi L. Spreng)

Identification

It is low lying, trailing shrub that generally grows prostrate with leaves that are evergreen, dark, and leathery and spatula-shaped or Obovate. The alpine variety produces larger leaves, the fruit is a red berry and it is also known as bearberry or Kinnikinnick.

Habitat

Is found in dry as well as boggy areas. The plant often grows at the base of trees such as juniper, tamarack, pines, etc.

Edible

The berries are red, mealy, dry, and do not have any flavor, so they need to be cooked with ingredients that have strong flavors to make them palatable. Berries are dried and smashed to form a flour-like meal. The Bella Coola Nation people mixed the berries with fats and consumed them while the Lower Chinook peoples mixed the dried berries with fat to make them edible. The berries are added to various stews and soups. Sauté the berries in grease and then mash them. Add this mash to fish eggs and sweeten to taste.

Uses

Traditionally the infusion of the whole plant was used to make a salve to treat sores, rashes, and similar problems. A lot of things go into this salve, including grease from animals and glue from animal hooves. The aerial parts are used to make an infusion that can be used as a mouthwash to treat sore gums and canker sores. Dried stems and leaves can be made into a powder that can be used as a poultice on wounds. An infusion made with stems, berries, and leaves can be ingested orally for bladder problems and to clean the kidneys. This infusion can also get rid of back pain and certain sprains. The Kwakiutl people smoked the leaves for their narcotic effects. It also has diuretic and astringent properties.

In Modern medicine, the plant is recommended for various problems of the urinary tract. Commercially it is available in various forms, including tea, powder, capsules, etc. It is frequently used in homeopathy. The tea is considered to be an astringent, styptic, diuretic, and antibacterial. The tea can be used internally as well as externally for its anti-inflammatory and antimicrobial properties.

Caution

Do not use if you are nursing or are pregnant. Do not eat acidic foods when using the tea, especially if you are using the tea to treat urogenital and biliary tract problems. It should not be used by children and people who suffer from high blood pressure. Prolong or excessive use of the plant can deal with damage to the liver and may also irritate the kidneys and bladder.

Wintergreen

Ericaceae (Gaultheria procumbens L.)

Identification

It is a small and evergreen forest that spreads using adventitious roots. The leaves are oval, evergreen, and glossy. The flowers are shaped like drooping bells and are white and waxy. The fruit is white when raw and red when ripe. It is also known as Canada tea, teaberry, or checkerberry.

Habitat

It is generally found in the Northern states of the United States of America and Canada. It normally grows around the base of trees but can also be found in open areas.

Harvest

The leaves should be harvested when tender. The berries are hard to find but should be harvested when ripe.

Edible

The plant is used to make delicious and calming wintergreen tea. The leaves can be chewed on as well. The berries are not found frequently as forest creatures often consume them. The plant has a delicious and unusual flavor that changes when it is dried. This is why it is recommended to try both the fresh-leaf tea and the dry-leaf tea to experience the two distinct tastes. Wintergreen is also used to add scents to candles and as a flavoring agent in gums. The tea can be used as a gargle to treat sore throat.

Uses

Traditionally it is believed that the plant has diuretic, astringent, lactagogue, and emmenagogue properties. The leaf tea was used to treat fevers, stomachaches, colds, kidney ailments, headaches, and dysmenorrhea. The tea was used topically to reduce muscle aches and rheumatism.

In modern use, wintergreen oil is not used as much as it is used in traditional medicine. It is sometimes added to liniments and ointments used to treat sciatica and neuralgia. The oil is astringent and antiseptic.

Caution

Avoid overuse. Excessive oral and subcutaneous doses can prove to be fatal. As little as 4 grams of the essential oil can be toxic or even fatal. The oil can also cause severe allergies. Pregnant women should avoid using tea or oil as it has uterine-stimulating properties.

Celandine

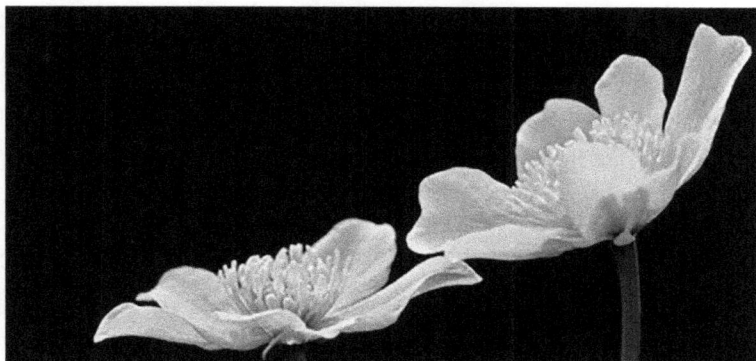

Papaveraceae (Chelidonium majus L.)

Identification

It has deeply cleft, poppy-like leaves with hairy petioles. The flowers generally have four petals, are yellow colored and look like poppy flowers. It is also known as wood poppy, celandine poppy, and greater celandine.

Habitat

It grows well in a rich, shady, and moist atmosphere. It requires well-drained soil. It can be found in Ohio, Michigan, Minnesota, Illinois, and other states in May. If you move north, the blooming periods differ.

Not edible

Harvest

The leaves and roots can be harvested upon maturation.

Uses

The Iroquois used this plant along with milk to sedate pigs. The orange color sap is used to treat warts, scabies, edema, etc. and the root was chewed in the past to treat toothache. It can be used internally to soothe various liver problems, including problems related to gallbladder, bile ducts, hepatitis, and jaundice. It is considered to be a uterine stimulant, anti-inflammatory, antispasmodic, circulatory stimulant, diuretic, and laxative. It was used in traditional Chinese medicine to treat irregularities related to menstruation.

In modern medicine, the plant is still used to treat gallbladder and liver problems. An infusion of the whole plant is used to treat inflammation, constipation, and to improve the flow of bile. It can also help the reproductive and circulatory systems. It is a liver stimulant that can treat inflammation of bile ducts and gout. It is a bitter-tasting plant, and it can stimulate the appetite.

According to certain sources, it can also treat rheumatism, arthritis, fever, bronchitis, coughs, etc. It can be used internally to treat ulcers. Externally nowadays, many dermatologists use it to wash ringworms, warts, psoriasis, eye inflammations, sores, etc. A lot of independent research is required to confirm more of these properties.

Club Moss

Lycopodiaceae (Huperzia lucidula [Michx] Trevisan; H. selago L.)

Identification

It is a miniature, low-lying plant that is around 10" tall. It is found under conifers and hardwoods in colonies. The leaves are evergreen and lance-shaped, the stems are vegetative and forking. The spores are seen in the sporangia shaped like kidneys.

Habitat

It is found throughout the world in moist forests and atmosphere. Generally, it grows under trees. Some people consider it to be a native of China or Eastern Europe.

Not Edible

Uses

Native Americans use it as a remedy for cold, a blood purifier, and for various topical and dermatological purposes while the Iroquois uses it to boost the immune system. H. selago is purgative, cathartic, emetic, and can improve immunity, especially during menstruation. Traditionally it was used to treat headaches by applying on the eyes in the form of a poultice. In modern times its antiviral components and chemistry is being studied. According to some speculative studies, it can prove to be beneficial against HIV. The infusion has a diuretic effect. Many homeopathy practitioners use it to treat problems of gallbladder, liver, respiratory problems, blood poisoning, inflammation of the female genitals, and other similar inflammations.

Caution

Consult a health practitioner before using the product.

Lady's Slipper Orchid

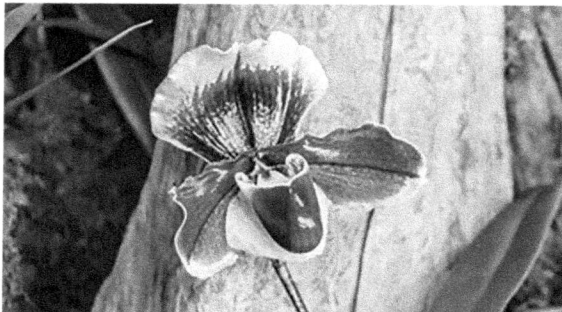

Cypripedioideae (Cypripedium acaule Aiton)

Identification

A dazzling perennial beauty with basal, lily-like, lance-shaped, stalkless leaves that can grow up to 10". They are bright green on the top and pale on the bottom. The horizontal rhizome produces pink (and in rare cases, white) slipper-shaped orchid-like flowers. The fruit capsules are brown.

Habitat

It is generally found in wet black spruce sites and Northern and Upland pine forests but can also be found in open wetlands. It is found in large numbers in southern Ontario and Northeastern states. Grows in abundance on the north shore of Lake Superior.

Not Edible

Harvest

Harvest the rhizome once the blooms have died out, i.e., in autumn.

Traditional Uses

The root i.e., the rhizome, is full of medicinal properties. It is astringent and styptic and is considered to be a tranquilizer, which has led to overharvesting. The rhizome was used as a tincture or decoction by the Native Americans for a variety of purposes, including cramps, colds, nervousness, menstrual problems, hysteria, flue, diabetes, inflammations, and spasms. The rhizomes harvested in autumn can either be used fresh or can be dried to use later. Due to the shape of the flower, this plant was considered to be one of the best aphrodisiacs. It is a protected plant because it was overharvested to the legal use of this plant is no longer allowed and has been discontinued. It is still used to treat insomnia and anxiety, although the chemical compounds have not been studied.

Caution

Handling the pink lady's slipper may lead to contact dermatitis.

Black Cohosh

Ranunculaceae (Actaea racemosa L. Nutt.)

Identification

It is a medium-sized perennial with the tough, knotty, and dark-colored rhizome. The leaves are smooth, double pinnate, and serrated. The flowers are drooping and can have three to eight petals. The sepals hide the bud of the flower.

Habitat

It is generally found in southern Canada and Eastern states of the United States of America.

Not Edible

Harvest

The rhizome contains the medicinal properties. It should be harvested either before blooming or after it.

Uses

Root infusions were used to promote lactation, induce abortion, and stimulate menstruation once upon a time. An infusion made with roots and alcohol was used to treat rheumatism. The infused root was used as a blood purifier, as a tonic, and a stimulating decoction. The pulverized roots can be added to the bathwater to reduce the pain of arthritis. The extract of the plant is still used to treat menopausal problems and premenstrual syndrome.

Many commercial preparations used to treat menstrual pain, cramps, uterine spasm, hot flashes, vaginal atrophy, mild depression, and menopause include extracts of black cohosh. As stated above, it has an estrogenic effect that brings down the luteinizing hormone levels.

According to a study, the extracts can be used to reduce psyche disturbances and hot flashes in menopausal women. People who have breast cancer can use the extracts to reduce sweating, hot flashes, and other similar problems, including insomnia and anxiety- all side-effects of premenopausal breast-cancer treatment. It also increases bone formation in postmenopausal women. Many holistic professionals use the plant to treat insomnia, fever, and arthritis.

Caution

Do not use without consulting with a proper holistic health-care professional, especially if you plan to use it for hormone replacement therapy, dysmenorrhea, and/or menopausal symptoms. Do not use it if you are lactating or are pregnant. The MHRA i.e., the United Kingdom health-care products regulatory and EMEA i.e., the European Medicines Agency have both warned patients to stop using the plant immediately if they see signs of liver toxicity. Those signs include loss of appetite, tiredness, blood in urine, stomach pain, vomiting, nausea, dark urine, yellowing of eyes and skin, etc. In the

United Kingdom, the manufacturers must add a warning about black cohosh on the label of the product.

Blue Cohosh

Berberidaceae (Caulophyllum thalictroides L. Michx.)

Identification

It is a leafy perennial that grows erect from a branched rhizome. The leaves are ovate and tri-pinnate, are finely divided and have three lobes. The flowers arise from the terminal leaf, have six sepals and can be purple or yellowish-green. Each over contains two dark-blue seeds. This plant is also known as papoose root or squaw root.

Habitat

It is found in wet woods in the states of Arkansas, South Carolina, Iowa, Minnesota, etc.

Not Edible

Uses

It is used in ethnic black medicine and Native American Medicine to facilitate childbirth. It is supposed to have a diuretic and analgesic effect and was consumed orally by the Cherokees for its antirheumatic and anticonvulsive properties while the crushed leaves were used to treat poison ivy and poison oak. The Chippewa used the decoction of the scraped roots as an emetic. Many tribes use their extracts to reduce excessive menstruation. The Mohegan and

Meskwakis use the herb to treat urinary and kidney problems and the decoction can also be used as a sedative. In modern medicine, the rhizome is used to make liquid extracts that can be used to treat gynecological disorders. The extract has an estrogenic effect and is used to treat uterine spasms, potential miscarriage, and dysmenorrhea. The Chinese use the extracts to treat external wounds. They also use the decoction to treat hepatitis and bronchitis.

Caution

The drug has uterine and heart stimulating effects and should not be used with proper medical guidance. It is recommended to use blue cohosh only with the advice of a skilled holistic health-care practitioner. Do not use this plant if you are pregnant or have heart diseases, disorders, or hypertension.

Black Nightshade

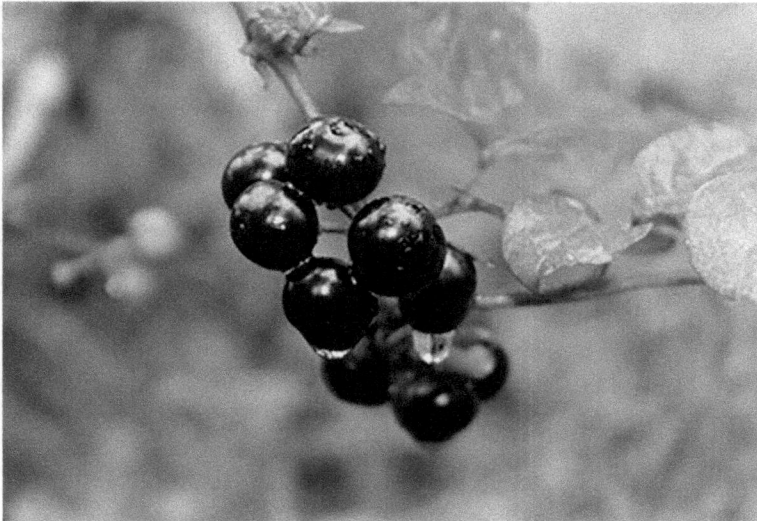

Solanaceae (Solanum nigrum L.)

Identification

It is a medium-sized, erect perennial with multiple branches and an abundance of leaves. The leaves are round to ovate and fleshy and can be either smooth or hairy. The white flowers bloom in fall. The flowers have five stamens, and they grow in groups of six or more blossoms. The fruit is green, yellow, or blackberry.

Habitat

It is found throughout the world in forests, fields, roadsides, etc.

Harvest

Harvest the berries when ripe.

Edible

Cherokees consumed it as a potherb. The berries and fruit were used to make pies, preserves, etc. Many plants that belong to the nightshade family i.e., the Solanaceae family, are considered to be toxic, but others are perfectly edible, including potatoes, tomatillos, tomatoes, and peppers. Do not consume an unknown species without consulting an expert.

Uses

The juice of the berry was used to treat tumors. The berries are considered to be diuretic. The juice of the plant was used as an emollient and laxative. Native Americans used this plant as an emetic. The decoction was used as a poultice or wash for wounds and skin problems such as hemorrhoids, psoriasis, and eczema. The smoke of the dried plant, when inhaled, can treat toothache.

In modern medicine, S. nigrum is used to make preparations that have anti-inflammatory, diuretic, antitumor, antioxidant, liver protectant, and immune modulator, properties. It can also reduce fever. Ayurveda experts believe the berries to have aphrodisiac properties. Black nightshade is available in the form of liquid, powdered, dried, and cut extracts. The moistened plant can be used as a rinse or a compress. Internal use needs to be monitored by a holistic health-care professional. The plant extracts are used internally as well as externally in traditional Chinese and Indian medicines.

In Ayurveda, the plant is thought to be a panacea. It is used for a variety of purposes including to treat bronchitis, asthma, dysentery fever, congestive heart failure, heart disease, hiccups, and inflammation. It is also used for its laxative properties and as a tonic. The dried fruits can be used as alternative and diuretic.

Caution

Do not use it without proper medical supervision.

Ginseng

Araliaceae (Panaxginseng C.A. Meyer; P. quinquefolius L.; Panax trifolius L.)

Identification

It is a medium-sized perennial with a round and smooth stems. The leaflets are finely serrated. The flowers are greenish-yellow, which produces glossy seeds the size of peas. The dwarf variety is similar to the regular variety but is smaller.

Habitat

It is found in the wild in Eastern and Northwest forested areas. It is a rare herb but is cultivated throughout the country. It needs well-drained soil with a mature, shaded canopy.

Harvest

The roots should be harvested when the plants are mature. This may take around a couple of decades.

Uses

The roots of the plant were used by the Native Americans to keep the ghosts away. Traditionally the decoction made using dried or fresh roots was used to induce sweating and reduce fever. The root is considered to be a panacea in Korea and China, where it is used as an overall tonic. The root is considered to be an aphrodisiac and can enhance immunity. It can also improve blood pressure and blood sugar levels. In Traditional Chinese Medicine, it is used to tone the primordial energy. It is also used as a tonic for the lungs in the spleen.

Ginseng has a multitude of uses in modern medicine too. According to the research conducted by Korea, China, Russia, and Europe, ginseng increases the production of interferon. It can improve endurance and is an ergogenic aid. It can regulate plasma glucose. A lot of research is going on about its antiproliferative, anticancer, and antitumor properties, especially against lymphoma, and leukemia. It has antifungal and antimicrobial properties. The preparation made using the roots of ginseng can be used to control the levels of blood pressure. Ginseng can also resist infection. According to certain studies, it can also improve mental acuity. Some studies suggest that it can prevent and protect the user from radiation sickness, and various other chemicals, physical, and biological stresses. It is perhaps the closest 'heal-all' herb in nature.

Asian ginseng (P. ginseng) is stimulating and 'warming.' Korean red ginseng is more warming than Asian, white ginseng. American ginseng (P.quinquefolius) is cooling, and it soothes and moistens. It is believed that ginseng has performance-enhancing effects, but these effects have not been tested yet.

Caution

Do not use this herb without consulting with a doctor. Strict supervision is necessary. Using more than three grams of ginseng per day can lead to insomnia, diarrhea, dermatitis, and anxiety. Some mild side-effects include skin rashes and headaches. Ginseng can boost the effects of caffeine but large doses may lead to asthma-like symptoms, hypertension, and heart palpitations. In rare cases, it may even lead to menstrual problems such as dysmenorrhea. Do not use ginseng if you have a fever, diabetes, hypertension, emphysema, upper respiratory tract infections, arrhythmia, bronchitis, and asthma. Never use it if you are on steroid therapy. Do not use during pregnancy or nursing.

Notes

Ginseng has become rare in the wild and should not be harvested frequently. It is better to buy them off trusted sellers and reputed markets.

The Chinese herbs often contain larvae and eggs of exotic insects and beetles, which is why all the roots imported from china are now sprayed with fungicide. Scrub the roots clean before using them. The roots can be excessively hard, so used strong grinders only.

Goldenseal

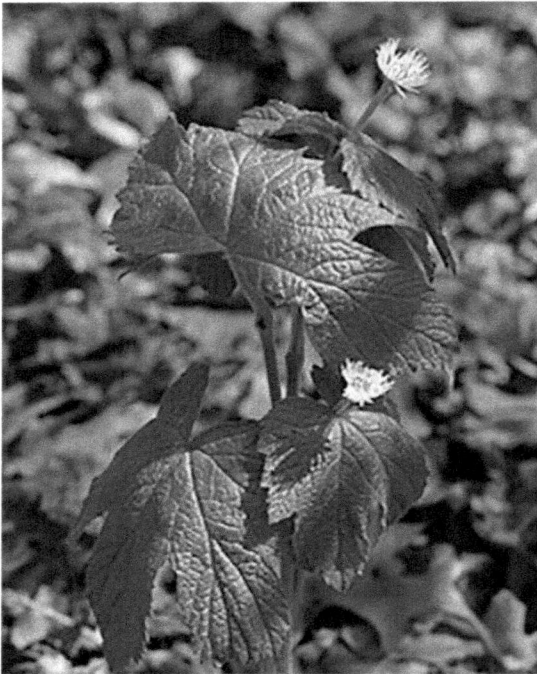

Ranunculaceae (Hydrastis Canadensis L.)

Identification

It is a perennial plant that produces golden or bright yellow rhizome. The leaves are ribbed and serrated. The flowers are single and grow on an erect stem while the fruit is scarlet and may produce a couple of glossy seeds. It spreads profusely and grows in dense colonies.

Habitat

It is found in abundance in Eastern parts of the USA. It grows in forests and needs well-drained soil and generally grows around ginseng. It can also be cultivated.

Harvest

The rhizomes can be harvested upon maturation.

Uses

Air-dried rhizomes are used to treat diarrhea. The decoction made using roots was used by the Cherokees to treat cancer and as a wash for infections, inflammations, and wounds. Goldenseal is also used to treat dyspepsia and an appetite stimulant. The dried root can be chewed to get rid of whooping cough while the filtered decoction can be used as eyewash and treatment for earache. Traditionally the root steeped in whiskey was used as a heart tonic. The extracts from the roots were used to treat liver problems, scrofula, tuberculosis, and gall problems traditionally.

In modern medicine, the dried root hair and rhizomes can be taken with water to stimulate the secretion of bile and hydrochloric acid. It can improve peristalsis. The drug shows slight antineoplastic and antibiotic properties. It can cleanse and stimulate the liver and can be used to constrict the peripheral blood vessels. It is used to treat upper respiratory tract infections. According to traditional Chinese medicine, the internal ingestion of goldenseal can increase white blood cell count. It provides a quick and easy remedy against travelers' diarrhea. The paste of root can be used to treat fungal infections and wounds. Goldenseal has a bitter taste, which is why it is often used to treat anorexia and to stimulate hunger. If you buy over-the-counter products, please consult a doctor or read the instructions carefully before using it.

Caution

Do not use if you are pregnant or nursing as it has uterine-stimulating properties. There is little to no research available on the effect of the plant on breast milk and the secretion of alkaloid. Goldenseal is excessively bitter, which is why some individuals may reject it. Proper dosages are nontoxic, but large dosages contain physiologically active chemicals such as hydrastine and berberine, which can prove to be fatal. Excess therapeutic dosages may lead to nervousness, stomach problems, and even depression while large doses may lead to involuntary reflex action, hypertension, convulsions, respiratory failure, and in extreme cases, paralysis and death. The herb may stop the activity of heparin.

Notes

It is difficult to find goldenseal in the wild because of overharvesting. Nowadays, it is cultivated widely can be found in stores easily.

Skullcap

Lamiaceae (Scutellaria baicalensis; S. lateriflora L.)

Identification

This is a perennial plant with oval to lance-shaped leaves that are toothed. The flowers are bluish-violet, hooded, and lipped. They grow from leaf axil on racemes.

Habitat

They are generally found in the East of Mississippi across the west and in Oregon. This plant grows abundantly in thickets, mature woods, etc. .

Not Edible

Uses

The Cherokees used S. lateriflora to promote menstruation and to treat dysmenorrhea. A decoction made with the plant was used to reduce after birth pain. Powdered root infusion was used as a throat and mouthwash. Traditionally the tea made with S. lateriflora's was used to treat rabies with great success. The tea contains antispasmodic and sedative properties.

In modern medicine, it is generally used to treat diarrhea and dysentery. It has positive effects on the liver as it contains anti-inflammatory bioflavonoids. S. barbata is used as a detoxifying agent for the liver.

Caution

Do not use it without proper medical supervision. Unspecified doses can be toxic.

Mistletoe

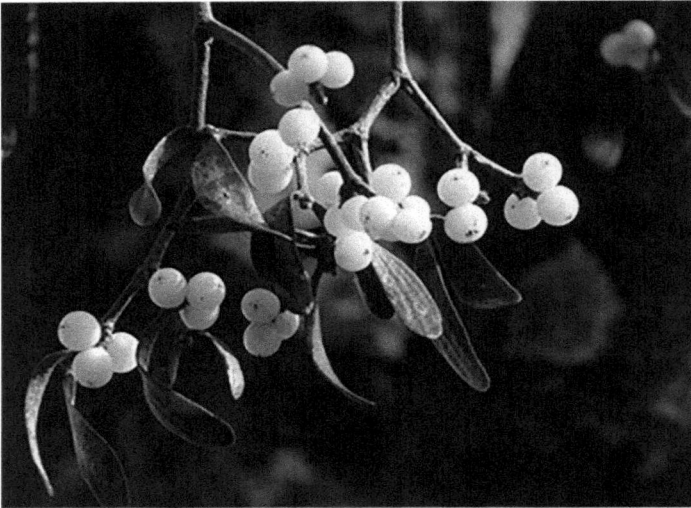

Santalaceae (Phoradendron tomentosum; also called P. Macrophylla [Engelm.] Cockerel)

Identification

It is a semi-evergreen, thickly branched, parasitic epiphyte that grows on the branches of valley oak, blue oak, and other oak trees. The leaves are ovate to oblong. It is also known as injerto.

Habitat

It is found between the areas of Texas to California and can be commonly found in plantation gardens, wooded roadsides, yards, etc. It is seen on hackberry, mesquite, oak, ash, willow, cottonwood, and sycamore trees.

Not Edible

May Cause Dermatitis

Uses

Mistletoe is dangerous, and many women have died in the past to use it to induce abortion. European pagans used V. album for its aphrodisiac properties (unproven). Native Americans considered this plant toxic (it is). In modern times the plant is being researched for its potential anti-diabetic properties. The extract is used by doctors to treat rheumatism. Its effects on cancer are being studied as well. The V. album variety can be effective against diarrhea, asthma, nervousness, tachycardia, whooping cough, amenorrhea, and epilepsy.

The plant should not be used unless explicitly prescribed by a doctor.

Caution

All parts of the plant are toxic. Multiple people have died in the past by consuming the berry tea. Only use it for decorative purposes during Christmas and contact a health professional immediately if you consume it accidentally.

Ground Nut

Fabaceae (Apios Americana medicus L.)

Identification

It is a twining and climbing perennial that grows like a pea vine. It has multiple tubers. The leaves are compound and alternate. The flowers grow in clusters and are generally purple, pink, or red-brown.

Habitat

It grows well under shade on wet grounds around the fringes of bogs, streams, thickets, etc. It grows profusely in deep, shady, and marshy areas. It can be found throughout the United States of America except in lower Florida, southern California, and extreme deserts.

Harvest

The seeds and tubers can be harvested upon maturation.

Edible

Seeds and tubers are edible. The seeds can be cooked like lentils. The tubers are full of protein and can serve as a great substitute for potatoes.

Uses

The Native Americans used the seeds as survival food. Most of the eastern tribes consumed the roots and seeds without which they would have starved in the winters. It can bring down cholesterol and maintain blood sugar levels. It is a hardy perennial that you can grow in your garden as well.

Indian Cucumber

Liliaceae (Medeola virginiana L.)

Identification

The plant has lancelet to ovate leaves that grow in a whorl around the stem. The plant grows around the base of hardwood trees. The root needs to be dug out to harvest the 'cucumber.'

Habitat

The plant prefers old-growth and grows well in deciduous and moist forests. It is often found growing under the hardwoods such as oaks.

Harvest

The plant needs to be dug out to harvest the 'cucumber.'

Food

The root tuber of the plant is edible, and it tastes like cucumber. It should be cleaned thoroughly and eaten raw.

Uses

Traditionally the Native Americans treated the plant as a panacea. The infusion made with the whole plant was used for a variety of skin problems. The berries were used for their anticonvulsive properties and the tea made from the root has diuretic properties. Traditionally Iroquois used the dried berries to treat convulsions in infants.

The traditional uses are still being employed all over; however, they have not been proved yet.

Wild Ginger

Aristolochiaceae (Asarum canadense L.)

Identification

It is a colonial and perennial herb that has an aromatic root that gives out the smell of ginger. The leaves are heart-shaped and dark green. The stems and leaves are hairy. The flower is red and generally blooms in May. The plant propagates through an adventitious rhizome. It spreads profusely.

Habitat

Many different varieties grow all over the United States of America except in lower Florida, southern California, and extreme deserts. It is found in moist woods and needs rich soil and shady areas.

Edible

It is technically edible but not eaten often. The roots can be boiled until tender and then drizzled with maple syrup and the crushed roots can be added to salads as a dressing. The dried and grated roots can be used as a substitute for Asian ginger.

Uses

The root was used to treat cough, colds, etc. It was also used as a tonic thanks to its antiseptic properties. It was combined with certain herbs to treat nervousness, scarlet fever, sore throat, headaches, vomiting, earaches, and other similar problems, including convulsion and asthma.

In modern medicine, the root is used to stimulate the appetite. The tincture is used by herbalists to dilate peripheral blood vessels, but more study is required.

Chapter 4

Herbs Found in Wetlands

These are generally soft-tissue plants that are found in low-lying areas such as marshes, rivers, wetlands, bogs, streams, lakes, and fens. Some of these can be found throughout the country.

American Lotus

Nelumbonaceae (Nelumbo lutea Wild.)

Identification

This plant is often confused with water lilies. It is a perennial plant that spreads by fleshy rhizomes as well as seeds, which is why it spreads far and wide. The flowers are generally yellowish to yellow and are 10" across. They generally have more than twenty petals and have an 'inverted shower-head' seed hold in the center. The leaves are round and bluish green and can be huge. Some leaves may stand above the surface of the water upon maturation with the help of rigid stems.

Habitat

It is a sun and water-loving plant which is found in abundance in the south, in Florida, and anywhere else where there is no current. They can also be found on Spring Lake in Illinois. They can be found east to the coast, south of the Rockies, and in California as well. In South America, they can be found as far below as Columbia.

Harvest

Multiple parts of the American lotus can be harvested for a variety of purposes. The shoots, roots, young seeds, and flowers can all be harvested once the plant starts to bloom. The seeds should be harvested when dry. The stem of the plant can be used for food as well.

Edible

Lotus is considered to be a vital source of food for Native Americans who eat shoots, roots, young seeds, and flowers. The root is full of calories and should be cooked before eating to remove/reduce bitterness. Unopened leaves can be eaten like spinach, or you can also use it as an edible wrap for various fillings. Stems are cooked in multiple ways. You can find Asian lotus roots in various markets where they are sold for food and medicinal purposes. The paste of seeds is used to make pastries and similar products. You can also boil the seeds, shell them, and eat them like peas.

Uses

Many Native American nations consider the American lotus to be a spiritual plant that has various mystic powers. It was (and still is) used by Ponca, Dakota, Omaha, Pawnee, and Winnebago for many different ceremonies. The roots were crushed and were used as a poultice for sores and wounds. The Asian relative of the plant is consumed for many different health benefits in its native land. Lotus has been a part of various cultures for thousands of years. It is found in various art forms, including sculptures, dance, music, and literature of India, Persia, Assyria, Greece, and Egypt. It is considered to be a sacred flower in India and forms an integral part of many different Ayurvedic medicinal formulas. In ancient Greece, it was considered to be a symbol of fertility, beauty, and eloquence.

In ancient Egypt, this flower was placed on the genital of female mummies.

Even in modern times, the flower is used for many different purposes, including medicinal. The Japanese suck the juice out of the stems by sucking out alcohol using the stems as a straw. In Asia, the seeds are consumed for the health of the heart, spleen, and kidneys. They are also used to treat infertility in men and diarrhea. The seeds have calming effects and can be used to get rid of insomnia and restlessness. The seeds contain alkaloids, which can help to lower blood pressure. The stamens of the flower are dried and used to make tea, which is good for the health of the liver. Lotus seeds do not expire easily, and dried seeds have germinated after hundreds of years too. Asian Americans frequently forage this plant.

Arrowhead, Wapato, Duck Potato

Alismataceae (Sagittaria latifolia Willd.)

Identification

The plant has a cleft, arrow-shaped leaves. The flowers generally have three petals. The plant has a deep-set tube that grows from a soft bottom. This plant is also known as Wapato or duck potato.

Habitat

It can be found along shorelines of lakes, edges of 'low-current' streams, lakes, ponds, etc. It is generally found in northern states such as Washington, Maine, etc.

Harvest

The tuber should be harvest in early spring or fall.

Edible

The tuber is considered to be a rich source of protein and starch. It is recommended to boil it until it becomes tender. Shell the skin and smash or sauté it. The tubers can also be roasted, peeled, and eaten out of hand.

Uses

The root is good for indigestion and some other stomach problems. The roots can be crushed and made into a poultice, which can be applied to abrasions, cuts, sores, etc.

American Pond Lily

Nymphaeaceae (Nymphaea Odorata Aiton)

Identification

It is a plant with large white flowers that can grow up to 5" across. The flowers have multiple petals, and the reproductive parts are yellow. The rhizomes are long and strong and are submerged in freshwater. The leaves are smooth and float over the surface of the water.

Habitat

These are generally found in still or gently moving, shallow waters. Often found in eastern and certain northern states. This plant is rare in Southwest but can be found in some places such as El Salvador.

Harvest

The leaves, buds, and flowers can be harvested when tender. The root is harvested upon maturation.

Edible

The leaves and buds are generally harvested in spring and cooked. They can also be eaten raw. Before using the flowers, wash the petals thoroughly as they generally have aquatic pests and larvae.

Uses

The dried roots can be sucked to treat mouth sores. The juice of roots is used to treat colds and similar problems. The roots are used for different purposes and in many different forms, including powder, juice, and decoction. It is generally used to treat coughs and colds.

In modern medicine, it is considered to be great homeopathic medicine for diarrhea. The root contains high amounts of tannin and is used to make a gargle to treat various diseases of the throat and mouth and to get rid of irritations and infections.

The decoction is used to treat many different vaginal conditions.

Notes

It is illegal to harvest this plant in a lot of states, so check with the department of natural resources before you try to harvest it.

Cattail

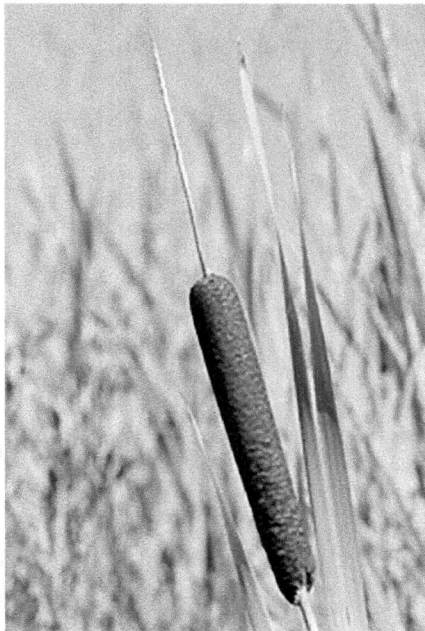

Typhaceae (Typha latifolia L.; T. Angustifolia L.).

Identification

It is a stunning perennial grass that grows up to 8' tall. It has lance-shaped leaves and has flowers that are shaped like two hotdogs. The upper 'hotdog' or head of the flower is male, while the lower one is female. Once the process of pollination is over, the upper head disappears after dispersal. Cattails are known for their large colonies and thus are widespread. Two commonly found species are Typha latifolia or the broad-leafed cattail and Typha angustifolia or the narrow-leafed cattail.

Habitat

It is found throughout the nation in shallow ponds, marshes, slow streams, and edges of lakes, wet grounds, and any wet and rich ground.

Harvest

The new shoots can be harvested in spring and summer, while the upper (male) head can be harvested in June. The roots can be harvested anytime.

Edible

The young and tender shoots are edible- just peel a few layers of leaves before using. The shoots can be sautéed in olive oil or butter. You can make simple meals by sautéing the roots and stir-frying them in olive oil. The male head can be used to add more starch to cornbread, bread, waffles, muffins, and pancakes. The male heads contain high amounts of essential amino acids, minerals, and vitamins.

Uses

The roots of Cattail are full of polysaccharides. The roots can be beaten into the water, and the remaining starch water can be applied over sunburn. The ashes produced by burning cattail leaves are antimicrobial and styptic and can be used to seal and dress wounds.

In modern medicine, the plant is no longer used for pharmaceutical uses. The water made by beating the roots can be used to boost the immune system, which can help you prevent many different acute infections, especially in the wilderness. The cattail is used to treat a variety of problems in the wilderness, especially for paddlers and trekkers.

Reed

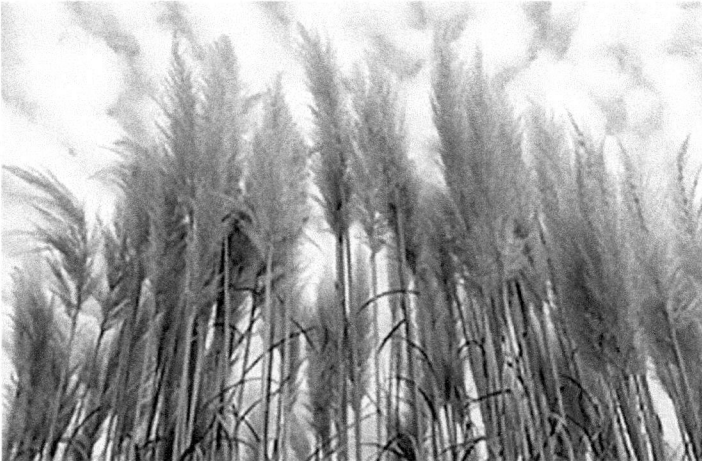

Poaceae (Phragmites communis L.)

Identification

It is a well-known and well-recognized grass that grows up to 9'. The roots are adventitious and grow just under the surface of the soil. The roots travel and send shoots wherever they go. The leaves are gray-green and lance-shaped. The flowers bloom in summer on the hollow stalk and in clusters. The flowers have 'hair' which moves in the wind swiftly. The flowers achieve their plumed shape in late summer when the seeds develop. The plant is also known as reed grass.

Habitat

There are multiple species found around the world. It mostly grows around marshes, wetlands, and lowlands.

Harvest

The shoots should be harvest in early spring. The seeds should be harvested in late summer.

Edible

Young and tender shoots are edible if harvested in early spring. Just remove the tough sheath-like skin of the leaves and chew on the white-colored, soft tissue underneath. The stalk can be chewed upon to get tender juices like sugarcane. The seeds are edible as well and can be added to oatmeal and other recipes, including bread and muffins.

Uses

Traditionally the decoction made with the roots can be used for analgesic effects. Traditional Chinese medicine uses two methods to make medicine using this plant. In the first method, the fresh root is soaked in rice wine until the roots absorb the wine. The plant is then dried and used in various decoctions to treat kidney, liver problems, insomnia, irregular menstruation, impaired hearing, tinnitus, frequent urination, diabetes, and allergies.

In the second method, the roots are steamed until they are black and then dried to make a decoction. This decoction is used to treat (although unproven yet) kidney, leukemia, constipation, hepatitis, diabetes, arthritis, internal bleeding, and rheumatism.

In modern medicine, the plant is crushed, and the juice is applied to stings and bites.

Duckweed

Lemnaceae (Lemna minor L.; L. gibba, and others)

Identification

It is one of the smallest flowering plants which grows as a hydroponic herb. It spreads by spreading a green floating cover over marshes, swamps, stagnant waters, lakes, etc. It's leaves look like the ears of Mickey Mouse. The threadlike root hairs soak minerals and waters from the pond. The green cover on the surface often looks like scum.

Habitat

It is found all over the nation floating gently on the surface of marshes, ponds, and still water.

Harvest

The leaves and roots can be harvested anytime.

Edible

The plant can be collected and dried to make tea. You can add fresh or dried duckweed to soups and similar recipes. Never eat this plant raw because it often comes from contaminated water sources. The plant has little to no taste. The plant generally contains small invertebrates like snails, which is why you should wash it carefully before using it. Use rarely and only when absolutely necessary.

Uses

Traditionally the whole plant is used as a warming agent in China to treat flatulence, hypothermia, inflammation, acute kidney infections, inflammation of the upper respiratory tract, jaundice, rheumatism, etc. The powder made from the whole dried plant can be used to make decoction and infusions. It was also used as a poultice by the Iroquois. In traditional Chinese medicine, it is used in combination with various herbs to treat epilepsy, acne, joint pain, and edema.

In modern medicine, the L. minor is used by homeopathic practitioners to treat fever, colds, and upper respiratory tract infections. Duckweed can also be used to treat yellow skin, liver problems, swelling of the upper airways, jaundice, etc. According to some practitioners, it can also be used to treat arthritis.

Gentian

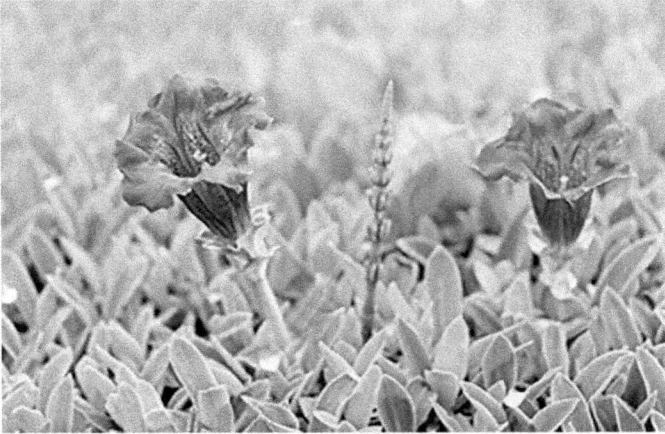

Gentianaceae (Numerous species: Gentiana andrewsii Griseb.;
G. crinite Froel. Ma)

Identification

It is a perennial plant that has clasping oval leaves with blue flower clusters. It is a stunning plant that may grow up to 30" but is generally shorter.

Habitat

Both the varieties of this plant are found in moist fields around wetlands, wet woods, and wet edges of old forests, and other similar places.

Not Edible

Harvest

The root can be harvested upon maturation.

Uses

Tincture and tea made with this herb are often bitter, which means they stimulate appetite and digestion. It was used by the Potawatomi to treat snakebite. It was used to treat backache by applying the boiled concoction of root and water. Traditionally, many people ate the roots and drank tea made using the aerial parts of the plant to stimulate appetite and help digestion.

In modern medicine, the herb is used as an effective bitter, and it used to stimulate the liver as well as the digestive system. It improves the processes of digestion, assimilation, and elimination and increases digestive secretions and peristalsis. The extract is easily available in health-food stores.

According to certain studies, the extract of Gentian lutea can also be used to treat diabetes; however, more research and trials are needed before any conclusive conclusion can be derived.

Lobelia

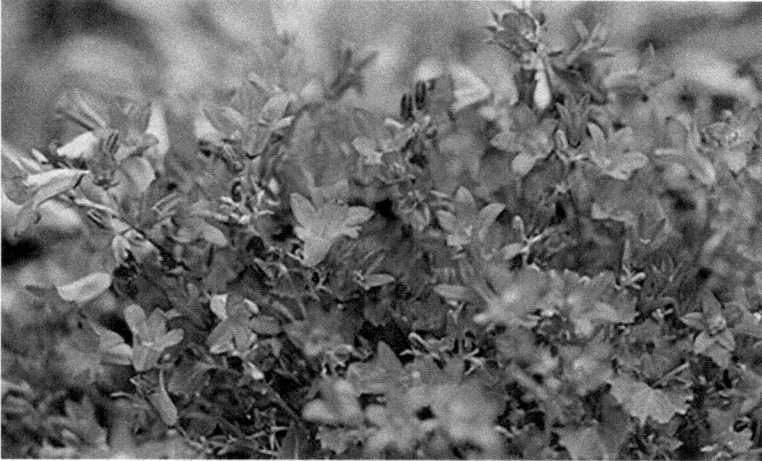

Campanulaceae (Lobelia siphilitica L.; Lobelia cardinalis L.)

Identification

The L. siphilitica variety is a perennial that grows up to 4" tall. The leaves are oval, while the flowers are generally blue or blue lavender white stripes. The flower looks distinctively like a bird.

Cardinal flower (L. cardinalis) looks like a bird, but it is not widely available, and instead of blue, it is red.

Habitat

There is a multitude of species, many of which are found from coast to cast. There are some subalpine species too. L. siphilitica is generally seen in moist areas, bogs, stream-sides, fens, and various other forms of wetlands. It is a predominantly southeastern and eastern plant, and it can be found even in Colombia, South America.

Not Edible

Harvest

Roots and leaves can be harvested upon maturation.

Uses

In traditional medicine, lobelia is used for a variety of purposes. It is used to increase respiration, induce vomiting, treat toothache, and as an analgesic as well. The L. siphilitica variety was used with Mayapple to treat sexually transmitted diseases. Many different species of lobelia have been used to treat cirrhosis, dysentery, gastroenteritis, eczema, edema, and schistosomiasis.

A poultice made with the roots of the plant can be used to soothe sore back and neck muscles. Both the leaves and roots can be used as an analgesic on stings, bites, sores, and boils, and also as a detoxifier. The plant can be used to make cold infusions, which are considered to be potent emetics. Lobelia has been used by a multitude of people to stop smoking, but if the practitioner is not an expert or is not skilled, they may lose their life. It has nervine and expectorant properties as well. The root is anthelmintic, analgesic, stomachic, and antispasmodic.

In the past, the tea made using the roots was used to treat syphilis, epilepsy, typhoid, cramps, stomachaches, worms, etc. The poultice of the routs was used to cover hard to heal wounds and sores. The leaves are febrifuge and analgesic. The tea made using the leaves of the plant can be used to treat nosebleeds, croup, colds, headaches, and fevers, along with many other things.

In modern medicine, many different alkaloids derived from various lobelia species have been patented, including lobelanidine, lobeline, lobelanine, etc. The alkaloids are extremely potent and are used to treat psychostimulant abuse along with various eating disorders. The above-mentioned drugs have been used to treat a variety of abuses, including amphetamines, cocaine, caffeine, barbiturates, opiates, cannabinoids, benzodiazepines, alcohol, hallucinogens, and phencyclidine. Many members of this family are being studied by various researchers all around the world for their efficiency against nervous disorders. According to a study conducted in 2012 and published in the Asian Pacific Journal of Tropical Medicine, it was found that extracts of lobelia halted the convulsions in epileptic mice

Caution

Do not use without expert and professional supervision. The plant is extremely potent and potentially toxic and can lead to a variety of problems.

Sweetgrass

Poaceae (Hierochloe Odorata L.)

Identification

It is grass with shiny, single stems that grow up to 18" to 20" tall. The base is violet-ish and is connected to the adventitious rhizome. The flowers are yellow, tulip-shaped, and adventitious. The leaves emit a sweet fragrance when crushed. It is also known as vanilla grass or holy grass.

Habitat

It is mostly found in the East along stream banks, moist meadows, and bog edges. It likes sunny locations. Native Americans cultivate it for ritualistic uses.

Harvest

Various parts of the plant can be harvested upon maturation.

Edible

In Europe, the grass is used to flavor vodkas and various liqueurs. The plant contains coumarin, which can aggregate antiplatelet, which may lead to excessive bleeding. The oil made from Sweetgrass (without coumarin) can be used to flavor soft drinks, candies, teas, alcoholic drinks, and perfumes. Tobacco chews are frequently flavored with this grass, and Native Americans often mix tobacco with the grass for smoking. The tea made using the leaves can be used to treat sore throat and coughs.

Uses

Many Indian nations throughout the country use this grass for spiritual cleansing and healing. The grass is burned, and smoke dispensed over people and places for cleansing. This process is known as smudging. The infusion can be ingested internally to treat coughs, sore throat, mouth problems, etc. The same infusion can be used externally as a wash for chafing, vaginal problems, and venereal diseases. In Europe, the grass is used in perfumes and other similar preparations.

In modern times, Sweetgrass is still used by many Indian nations in sweat-lodge ceremonies for purification and cleansing. The plant is considered to be a pliable and soft female plant which is supposed to bring in good spirits and make the soul fresh. The grass can also be weaved into baskets.

Caution

Do not use Sweetgrass internally as it contains a potent blood-thinning agent called coumarin.

Cranberry

Ericaceae (Vaccinium oxycoccus L.)

Identification

This is a short, evergreen shrub which generally grows like a creeper. It has a brown (sometimes black) colored bark, which is generally hairy but can be smooth too. The flowers are pink and generally grow solitary but can also be found in couplets and sometimes in three. The petals are bent backward, which makes them look like shooting stars. The fruit can be anywhere between pink to red. The berries are small and extremely tart and juicy.

Habitat

It is found in almost all states. It is found along the floor of sphagnum bogs, wet alpine meadows, in hummocks, and similar places.

Harvest

The fruits can be harvested when fresh and ripe.

Edible

Cranberries can be used in many different recipes and preparations. You can add them to turkey, apple crisps, pies, puddings, etc.

Uses

The berry juice and berries can be used to treat urinary tract infections as it is supposed to acidify urine. According to some sources, cranberry can be used to remove kidney stones. The juice can also be used to prevent urinary stones and to treat bladder infections. It contains high amounts of vitamin C and helps you prevent scurvy.

In modern medicine, it has been found that the juice can help you prevent the adhesion of Escherichia coli to the linings urinary tract, bladder, and the gut; this way, the bacteria do not multiply and keeps disease at bay. Cranberry juice is good for urinary system problems. The juice and the berries are used to reduce the degradation and odor of urine in incontinent patients. It can bring down the pH of urine by a significant amount, but more tests are necessary. It is recommended to talk to a professional before using the products for health-benefits.

Beach Wormwood

Asteraceae (Artemisia campestris L. subsp. caudata [Michx.] H.M. Hall & Clem.)

Identification

This plant has multiple species that are found throughout the world. It can either be a short-lived perennial, or it can be a biennial as well. In the case of biennial plants, the first year leaves are rosettes of grayish blue color. The second-year leaves are whitish green. The size of the leaves goes down upon the maturation of the plant. The leaves of the plant are hairy in the beginning but become smooth with maturation. The stems are light green to red and are branched. The young stem ends are matte and have fine hair. The hair disappears with the growth of the stem. It is also known as field sagewort or dune wormwood.

Habitat

It is commonly found in many different states of the United States of America. It is generally found in the dunes of the Great Lakes. If you are away from the dunes, look for sandy areas on the sides of the hills.

Edible

They are not used as food. The leaves of this plant are often used to make bitter teas, which can be used to treat indigestion. Certain species of Artemisia are also used to make absinth, which is used to flavor a variety of sprits, including vermouth.

Harvest

The plant can be harvested upon maturation.

Uses

The Tewa nation used the juice to treat upset stomachs and to relieve gas. The infusion of the leaves is also used to treat chills and fever. It has been used for thousands of years in a variety of traditional and holistic medicine schools. It is particularly popular in China and Europe.

It is still used in modern medicine. Artemisinin and thujone are anthelmintic, which means that they kill the worms present in the intestines. In Europe, it is a common practice to consume drinks made of Artemisia as a digestive aid or as stomach bitters. A synthetic derivative of Artemisia annua, artemisinin, is used to get rid of various parasites, including malaria. According to a recent study, it was found that artemisinin has a 97% success rate in most of the non-complicated cases of malaria.

Caution

Do not consume large doses of Thujone as it blocks the gamma-aminobutyric acid. This acid is essential, and if the production is blocked, it can lead to seizures and even death. Artemisia should not be consumed in large quantities as it can prove to be toxic.

Mint

Lamiaceae (Mentha spp.: M. Piperita L.)

Identification

Mint is one of the most commonly found and herbs all around the world. Many members of the mint family are found in the Americas as well. All the mints have certain similar characteristics, which include erect and squarish stem, aromatic leaves, etc. All mints spread aggressively. The height varies from species to species. The root is generally a rhizome that spreads around. The Leaves are elongated, roundish, serrated, and plump. The flowers are borne on terminal spikes are in dense clusters and whorls. The colors of the flowers vary according to species and can range from violet, white, blue, etc. Peppermint or Mentha piperita is the most commonly used species.

Habitat

M. Piperita can be found across the nation and is often found near stream banks, shorelines, and dunes of the Great Lakes, around avalanche slides, blowdowns, and wet meadows.

Harvest

The leaves and stalk can be harvested anytime throughout the growth period.

Edible

Peppermint has multiple uses in food. It can be used to flavor salads, teas, and cold drinks. It can be added to meat and vegetable preparations, curries, and other similar recipes and is an integral part of the Middle Eastern and South Asian cuisines. Ancient Romans used mint to flavor sauces and wines. Mint is great with chilled soups of all types and also adds a distinct flavor to Mexican bean soups.

Uses

Traditionally mint is used for many different purposes. Alexander the Great believed that drinking mint tea or eating the leaves led to unaggressive and listless behavior. Aristotle believed mint a potent aphrodisiac.

The flowers and leaves of the plant are used to make tea, which is considered to be uplifting. The tea (and extracted oil) has carminative, antiseptic, and warming properties. The tea can also relieve muscle spasms. The infusion can increase the secretion of bile and enhance perspiration. Peppermint contains two volatile oils called menthone and menthol, which are antiseptic, antibacterial, cooling, antifungal, and anesthetic to the skin.

In modern medicine, the extraction of the flower and leaves can be used to treat liver problems, dyspepsia, and gallbladder issues. The oil can be used to treat coughs, colds, fevers, bronchitis, mouth infections, larynx inflammations, dyspepsia, and liver and gallbladder issues. According to certain modern studies conducted in Europe, the extracts can also be used to treat IBS or irritable bowel syndrome. The oil and tea have an antispasmodic effect on the digestive system. Peppermint is also used to treat diarrhea, colic, flatulence, spastic colon, cramps, and constipation and headaches caused by digestive problems. Research is being made to find out the effects of peppermint on stress-related headaches, tension, and similar problems. The diluted oil can also be used for aromatherapy and to treat respiratory infections. It was found that peppermint can stop the growth of cells of laryngeal carcinoma and thus has anti-cancer effects.

Spearmint, peppermint, mountain mints, and other kinds of mints have edible leaves and flowers that can be added to desserts, salads, etc. It is a carminative herb that can be used to get rid of gas.

Caution

Do not use highly concentrated mint oil as it may irritate the skin and may even cause burns. Peppermint should not be used to treat gastritis, ulcers, and acid reflux as it relaxes the sphincter of the esophagus, which can lead to acid reflux.

Notes

If you plan to plant different kinds of mints in your garden, beware, mints spread aggressively, and often 'mate' with each other. These hybrids generally do not have a strong taste and medicinal properties. To prevent this, it is recommended to plant the mints away from each other and in good quality steel containers.

Watercress

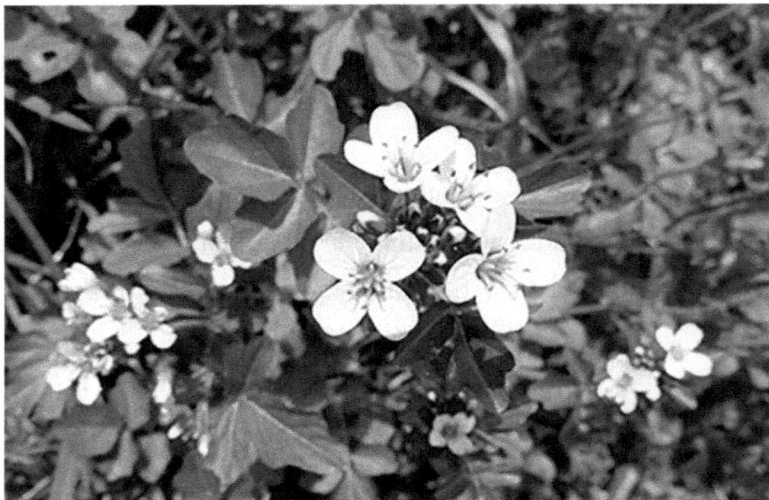

Brassicaceae (Nasturtium officinale L.)

Identification

It is a plant that loves water with floating mats and can rise to 14". The roots grow beneath the water. The stem is grooved and becomes fibrous and tough upon maturation and the leaves are alternate, paired, and ovate. The leaflets are broad towards the base. The flower is white and generally has four petals. It blooms mostly in May and may bloom throughout the year if the weather remains warm.

Habitat

It is found almost everywhere throughout the country, generally around temperate areas. It grows well near slow-moving streams and creeks. It also grows around springs and seeps.

Harvest

The leaves can be harvested when fresh. Do not harvest from random and unknown places.

Edible

Watercress belongs to the mustard family. It is pungent and spicy. Only harvest it from a clean and potable source of water. If you plan to use it raw, you must harvest it from your backyard or a similar source. The watercress can be uprooted and planted in the backyard with ease. Just keep it wet, and it will provide you an abundant harvest. It is one of the crucial ingredients of V8 vegetable juice. It goes well with Italian recipes.

Uses

It has been continuously used since ancient times. In fact, the father of medicine, Hippocrates, described it as a stimulating expectorant, a heart tonic, and a digestive. It is good for colds, coughs, and bronchitis. It can also help you to relieve gas. It is a diuretic and helps to clean the bladder and the kidneys. Mexicans use it as a spring tonic.

It contains a multitude of minerals, vitamins, and isothiocyanate. Eight ounces of the plant are added to the V8 cocktail. Studies are being done regarding its anti-cancer properties.

Horsetail

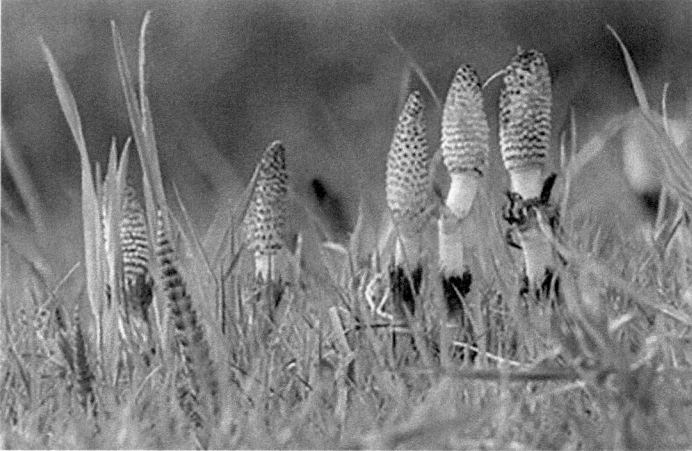

Equisetaceae (Equisetum hyemale L.; E. arvense L.)

Identification

It is perennial that can grow up to 5' in height. It grows in spring and looks like a naked segmented stem with a dry sporangium. If the plant is shaken, the spores fall off. After maturation, the plant becomes sterile, and a stem comes out with needle-like branches arranged in the shape of whorls. It is also known as equisetum or a scouring rush.

Habitat

It is found around bogs, fens, marshes, streams, rivers, and lakes throughout the country.

Harvest

The shoots can be harvested when young and tender.

Edible

Many Native Americans eat the tender shoots as a tonic. The Japanese boil the tips and eat them. They can also be mixed with vinegar, soy, rice, ginger, and other ingredients. The roots are edible too.

Uses

Traditionally, it was used by Mexican Americans to make various kinds of decoctions and infusions. They made decoction/infusion with aerial parts to treat painful urination. The plant contains a high amount of bioflavonoids and equisetonin, which is good for its diuretic effect. The stems of the plant can be crushed to form a poultice, which can be used to treat rashes in the groin and armpit. The Blackfoot Indians used the infusion of the stem as a diuretic. An infusion of the aerial parts of the plant was used by the Cherokees to treat coughs in their horses. The infusion can also be sued to treat backaches, dropsy, sores, and cuts. Bathing in the infusion was prescribed as a remedy for gonorrhea and syphilis. It is one of the most used herbs by the First Peoples.

In modern medicine, the extracts can be used internally to treat kidney and bladder stones along with urinary tract infections. The extract can be used externally to treat burns and wounds. It is available over the counter.

Caution

High amounts of the herb can prove to be toxic, which why it is necessary to use the herb only under the supervision of a licensed medical expert.

Notes

This is a quick-growing and fast-spreading plant which grows well in the sun and shade and can bring a fresh look to your flower garden. You can use the stems to clean pans and pots because of the high amount of silica.

Angelica

Apiaceae (Angelica atropurpurea L.)

Identification

It is a biennial with erect, thick, and purple stems. It has large, compound leaves which are divided generally into three to five leaflets that have hollow petioles. The upper leaves are covered with sheaths, which upon maturation collects at the base of the petioles. The flowers are greenish-white and look like umbrellas. It looks a bit like poison hemlock, which is why it is necessary to be cautious while foraging.

Habitat

It is generally found in the east of the Mississippi River. It is found along rivers, streams, and wet lowlands.

Harvest

The roots and leaves can be harvested upon maturation.

Edible

Traditionally not consumed. The roots are used as a flavoring agent for various jams, gin, vodka, and cooked fish.

Uses

The root of A. atropurpurea variety can be used to make decoctions to cure chills, rheumatism, flatulence, and fever. The decoction can be gargled to treat sore throat. It was often used in sweat-lodge ceremonies to treat headaches, arthritis, hypothermia, and frostbite. The crushed root can be used as a poultice to get rid of the pain. Both the varieties, i.e., A. Sinensis and A. atropurpurea, are used differently in Western and Asian traditions. Both plants have certain differences in their chemical composition too.

The A. Sinensis variety can be used as a warming tonic and is considered to be one of the topmost female herbs in the school of Chinese herbal medicine. It is used to reduce menstrual cramps and to increase the flow. It has antispasmodic properties and can reduce angina. Angelica contains calcium channel blockers- a property that is observed in commercial drugs that are used to treat angina. According to traditional Chinese medicine practitioners, the root can improve peripheral circulation.

In modern medicine, it is often used for a variety of purposes; for instance, German holistic professionals prescribe dried roots to treat indigestion and heartburn. European professionals use A. Sinensis to treat colic. Naturopaths from America use both the species, which is why it is recommended to contact a professional.

Balmony

Scrophulariaceae (Chelone glabra L.)

Identification

It generally grows in wetlands and produces showy white flowers with a slight pink tinge. The flowers generally bloom in late summers. The flower is long, two-lipped, and looks like snapdragon flowers or like the shell of a turtle. The leaves are shaped like a lance, are opposite with coarse teeth, and grow on dark green smooth stem. The seeds are bitter and round. Thanks to the appearance of the flower, this plant is also known as turtlehead.

Habitat

It is generally found in plains states, i.e., the Northeastern states. It is often found around boneset and Joe-Pye weed and it grows around lakes, bogs, and other similar moist areas.

Not Edible

Harvest

Harvest the roots after flowering.

Uses

Traditionally, the Cherokee used the herb to treat worms. The smashed roots were used to make anti-witchcraft potions. It was also used as an appetite stimulant thanks to its bitter taste. Many Native American nations use the herb as a laxative and to reduce fevers. The aerial parts are crushed to make an ointment, which can be used to treat painful breasts, ulcers, and inflamed tumors.

The aerial parts are used by homeopaths to treat various digestive and liver problems, especially worm infestation. Certain holistic practitioners still practice traditional methods of use.

Blue Flag

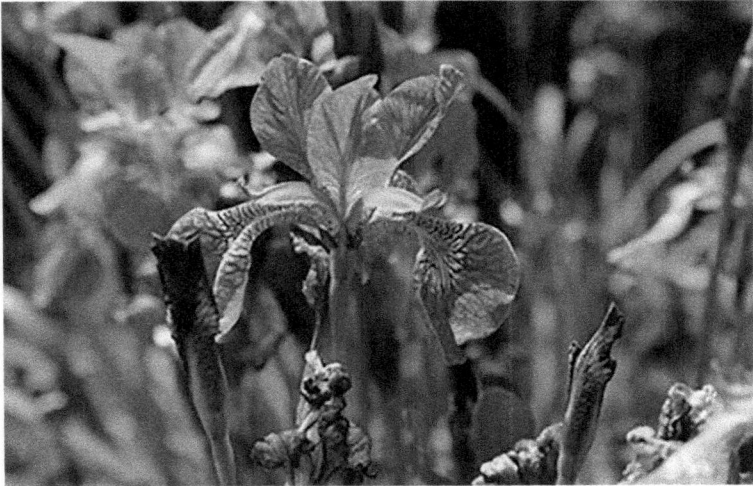

Iridaceae (Iris versicolor L.)

Identification

It is a perennial that grows up to 3' in height. It has sword-shaped, grayish-blue tinted leaves. The flowers are irregular, look like orchids, and are blue to violet. This plant is also known as the wild iris.

Habitat

It is widely distributed throughout the east of Mississippi and also in southern Canada. It is mostly found in fens, damp marshes, edges of lakes, and along streams. It can be transplanted to the garden and grows profusely.

Harvest

The rhizome can be harvested upon maturation.

Uses

The rhizome is poisonous, but it was used for its purgative properties by the Native Americans. It is cathartic, emetic, and diuretic. The root is used to make a decoction, which can be used to treat wounds and sores externally. It is ingested internally to treat cholera, colds, and earaches. The crushed roots are used as a poultice for wounds. The smashed roots are used to treat burns by the Algonquins. A poultice made with roots was used to treat sores, swellings, and scrofulous sores caused by tuberculosis by the Chippewas.

The root decoction is often used to treat kidney problems and arthritis. The Malecite people use the infusions to treat sore throat and similar oral problems. Other tribes often mix the smashed roots with flour and apply it to painful areas. The Omaha tribe people chew on the roots and then dip in its water and then let the juice drip in-ear to cure earache. The plant was thus viewed as a panacea by many communities and tribes.

It is used for a variety of purposes in homeopathic medicine. The rhizome and root hair can increase the production of bile and urine and are often used as a mild laxative. Blue flag is used to treat skin problems, indigestion, gallbladder, and liver problems. The herb stimulates the internal organs and has a detoxifying effect on the body and it is beneficial in constipation, skin problems, acne, eczema, etc. It can also be used to treat respiratory problems and headaches. Some people also use it as a weight-loss aid.

Caution

Overdose may lead to vomiting. Do not use it in pregnancy. The juice of the plant can irritate the digestive system and skin.

Jewelweed

Basalminacae (Impatiens capensis Meerb.)

Identification

It is an annual, fleshy succulent that grows in dense colonies. The stem is light green, simple, and looks almost translucent. It has swollen nodes. The leaves are ovate, thin, green, and generally have up to fourteen teeth. The flowers are small and are generally yellow-orange with brownish spots. They are irregular and spur-shaped. The fruit is a long capsule that bursts open when mature to spread seeds. This is why it is also known as spotted touch-me-not.

Habitat

It is commonly found in the east of the Rockies and can also be found sparingly in the west. It covers the ground densely in wetlands, lowlands, around lakes, fens, bogs, and streams.

Harvest

Harvest the flowers in summer and shoot sin spring.

Edible

The flowers can be consumed in the form of salads and stir-fries while the shoots can be added to soups, eggs, and various other vegetables and gravies. The flowers can also be used as a garnish.

Uses

The crushed aerial parts of the herb are used to treat poison ivy. It can bring down inflammation and itching if applied over the affected area. Native Americans used it to treat measles, dyspepsia, and hives. Infusion of the plant was used to treat congestive heart failure by the Creek Indians. The smashed flowers can be used to treat cuts, bruises, and burns.

The whole herb is infused to make a concoction that is diuretic and stimulant. Naturopaths generally use this to treat dyspepsia. It has anti-inflammatory properties and is used against poison oak, poison ivy, poison sumac, and many other similar conditions. It may not cure them, but it provides are soothing and cooling treatment.

Boneset

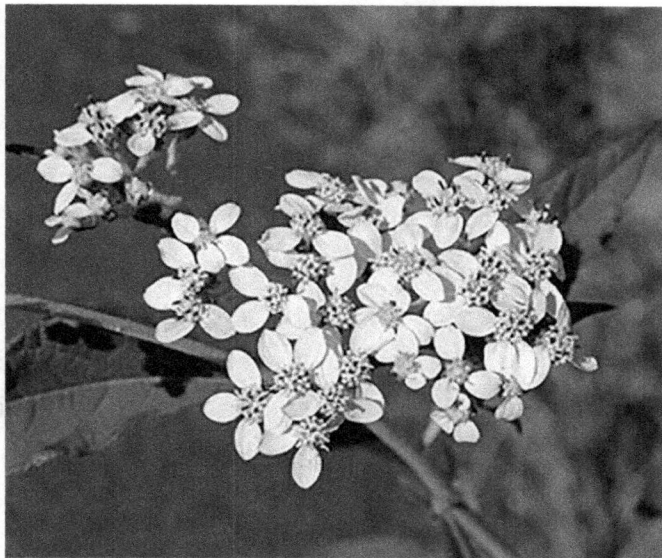

Asteraceae (Eupatorium perfoliatum L.)

Identification

It is a perennial plant that can grow up to 5' tall. It grows from a horizontal, hairy root-stock. The leaves and the stem are hairy too. The leaves are rough to touch, are shaped like a lance, and taper to a point near the stem. The white flowers bloom in florets at the top of the plant. Upon maturation, the plant makes tufted fruits.

Habitat

It is generally found in wetlands, thickets, marshes, and wet prairies in the Eastern United States.

Harvest

The leaves and roots can be harvested upon the maturation of the plant.

Uses

The tea made with leaf was used in the nineteenth century to break a fever, especially in the case of acute infections. The leaf tea stimulated the immune system and was used to treat malaria, colds, influenza, painful joints, arthritis, gout, pneumonia, and to induce sweating. The aerial parts of the plant can be crushed to make a poultice, which can be used to treat swellings, edema, tumors, etc. The Native Americans used the poultice made by crushing plants to set broken bones. The crushing plant can be used to make an infusion that can be taken internally. It is emetic and cathartic. The infusion can also be used to treat sore throat, stomach pain, hemorrhoids, headaches, etc. It can also reduce urinary problems and to reduce chills.

Homeopathic practitioners use microdoses of the plant to treat flu, colds, and other similar conditions. The dried aerial parts of the plant are used to make infusions, which can increase immunity. This infusion can be used to treat infections, colds, flu, and various other infections.

Caution

Micro-doses of the herb is diuretic and laxative. The larger doses can be used to induce vomiting and catharsis. The plant contains pyrrolizidine alkaloids. These dangerous compounds can prove to be toxic and can even destroy the liver. Do not use this plant without proper consultation from a licensed medical or holistic healthcare practitioner.

Joe-Pye Weed

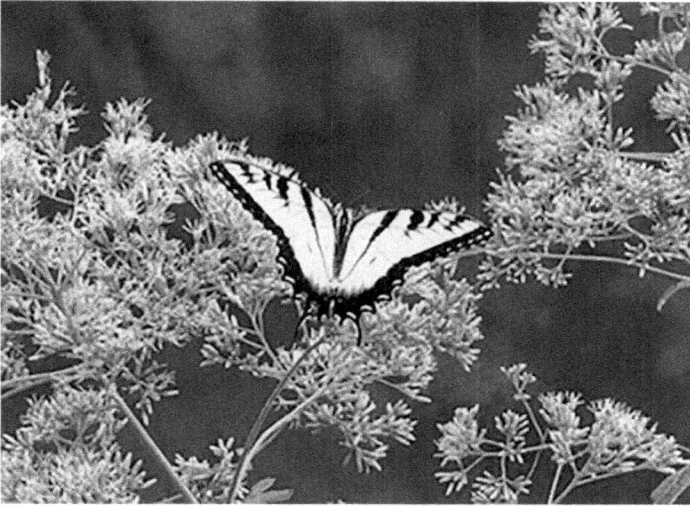

Asteraceae (Etrochium purpureum L. La Mont; E. maculatum L.)

Identification

It is a perennial that is found in the northern as well as southern states. In northern states, it grows up to 5' while in the southern; it can grow up to 10'. It has a stout stem that grows from a rhizome. The flowers are pink to purple can are shaped like disks. The leaves are shaped like a lance and grow up in whorls. Each leaf is toothed, hairy, and rough.

Habitat

It is generally found in eastern states of the United States of America and Canada. It grows in wetlands, marshes, fringes, lakesides, seeps and on Marsh, wetlands, fringes of wetlands, seeps, lakesides, and damp grounds.

Not edible generally. Certain American tribes use the ash made out of the root as a spice or a substitute to salt. The ash can also be used to make tea. The roots and aerial parts of the plant are used to make teas as well.

Harvest

The parts of the plant can be harvested upon maturation.

Uses

It is generally used by Native Americans to treat typhus and as revitalizing tonic. It has diuretic properties and can be sued to treat a variety of urinary tract problems. It can also be used as a relief against constipation. The tea made with the plant was used as a wash to inhibit infections and to promote healing. The root of the E. purpureum is supposed to be an aphrodisiac, especially Meskwakis, who sucked on the root while trying to woo a partner. The root decoction of the E. purpureum can be used to treat bed-wetting and dropsy. It was used to treat asthma, as well. The tea made using both the species was used by Native Americans to treat dysmenorrhea and menstrual disorders. It was also used as a recovery tea after pregnancy. The Cherokees used the tea made with E. purpureum to treat arthritis, rheumatism, and as a diuretic. The infusion of the root can be used as a laxative. Navajos believed that the root could be used as an antidote to many different poisons. The Potawatomi used freshly crushed leaves as a poultice.

In modern times aerial parts of the plants are used to make hot infusions by naturopaths to treat fever, colds, and arthritis. The plant can induce sweating and is an antimicrobial. It can also loosen phlegm and induce coughing to remove mucus. It can also be used as a laxative to get rid of worms from the body.

Caution

Pregnant and lactating people should not use this herb.

Bittersweet Nightshade

Solanaceae (Solanum dulcamara L.)

Identification

It is a climbing vine that has lobed, dark green, petioled leaves. The flowers look like rockets and are purple. The fruit appears in the fall and is blood orange. It is also known as climbing nightshade. It belongs to the family of tomato and potato.

Habitat

It can be found easily along ditches, streams, thickets, bogs, and lakeshores. It clings to shrubs and trees.

Not Edible

The berries are toxic and should not be consumed.

Harvest

Harvest the roots upon maturation.

Uses

Native Americans used the roots to make an infusion, which was used to treat nausea and gas. It was also used for its antiemetic properties. They used the extracts to make salves based on oil that was used externally. It is believed to have anti-cancer properties, but the effects have not been proven yet.

In modern medicine, it is used to treat eczema, acne, warts, and furuncles. In holistic medicine, it is used to treat gout, arthritis, and various respiratory problems, including cough and bronchitis. Contact a professional before using the herb.

Caution

The herb is toxic but rarely fatal. Do not take if pregnant or lactating.

Sweet Flag

Acoraceae (Acorus calamus L.)

Identification

It is a perennial plant that can grow up to 2' tall. It grows from a rhizome. The plant has a long stem with leaves that look like swords. The flowers are green and grow on a spadix that looks like clubs. The plant is extremely aromatic and grows in large colonies. The plant is also known as calamus.

Habitat

It generally grows on the east of Mississippi. It is found around creeks, wetlands, lakes, marshes, springs, streams, and seeps.

Not Edible

Traditional Uses

It is one the most used herbs for its potent medicinal properties and as a ritualistic plant too. The root is a sialagogue, which means that it makes the mouth water, which, as a result, makes the process of digestion easy. The Sun Dance ceremony is an important ritual where the First People may sing for ten hours or more. To keep the singing perfect, they tend to hold a piece of calamus root between their gums and cheek, which keeps the throats moist. Many Native Americans used garlands made out of sweet flag leaves to mask body odor.

The tea made using the roots stimulates appetite thanks to its bitter taste and aromatic nature. The infusion of the root was also used as a stomach tonic and to treat gastritis and dyspepsia. The root was chewed to treat toothache and it is believed to have sedative, nervine, and relaxant properties. The decoction was used to treat fevers, colds, coughs, congestion, and children's colic. The powdered and dried rhizome was inhaled as a remedy against congestion. It also has anticonvulsant, antispasmodic, and CNS (central nervous system) depressant properties.

In modern medicine, the peeled and dried rhizome is considered to be a tonic, carminative, stimulant, and antispasmodic. It increases sweating. In vitro studies say that it can also bring about anticlotting effects and can be used to treat impulsive and aggressive behavior. The extract is considered to have sedative and antispasmodic properties. The extract of the root is used as a remedy against gastrointestinal problems and to treat fungal problems. The Asian variety is considered to be an aphrodisiac. The strains found in the United States of America and Europe are used to treat ulcers. The A. Calamus var. americanus is often used to reduce stomach spasms and to relieve distended stomach and the headache associated with stomach ailments.

Caution

A. calamus contains Beta asarone. Over time, this compound has proven to be carcinogenic in animals; it is recommended to monitor the dosage properly. Do not use the herb for a long time. Avoid using unless prescribed, monitored, and guided by a licensed and skilled holistic healthcare professional. Always follow the instructions and dosage given on the package.

Chapter 5

Plants from Arid Zones
and Deserts

These the plants are generally found in the arid zones and the deserts in the United States of America. Most of these are found in the western states of the nation and Mexico. These plants do not require a lot of water and grow well in full sun.

Buffalo Gourd

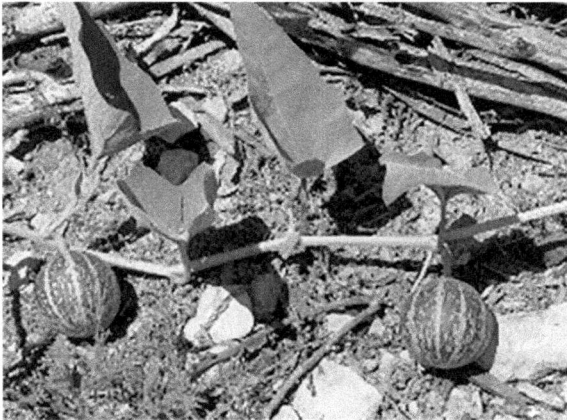

Cucurbitaceae (Cucurbita foetidissima Kunth)

Identification

It is an annual (and in some cases perennial) herb that has a hard stem thanks to calcium deposits. The stems have tendrils and are climbing. The stems are often branched with multiple tendrils. The leaves are rough, simple, hairy, palmately lobed, alternate, and veined. The flowers bloom through the nodes and are generally white to cream in color. The corolla is shaped like a cup and has five lobes. The fruit is medium-sized and looks like a melon or a gourd. It has a lot of seeds.

Habitat

It is generally found in semiarid areas and dry plains, especially in Southwest in states such as Arizona, Texas, New Mexico, Nevada, California, etc. It either sprawls on the ground or can also be found growing along the fences. Huge plants can cover up to 100 square feet ground or more.

Harvest

The seeds can be harvested upon the maturation of the fruit. The fruits and leaves can be matured when ripe.

Edible

The plant is bitter, especially the seeds, but they contain a high amount of protein. They become edible after cooking. The seeds are consumed only after they are dried and roasted. These procedures reduce bitterness by removing cucurbitacins or triterpenoid glycosides. High doses of these can be toxic. The seeds contain 35 percent protein and 43 percent oil, which makes them a great and economically viable crop. The seeds do not contain as many glycosides as the pulp of the gourd. This is why it is recommended to clean the seeds thoroughly before using them. The dried seeds can be cooked in an oil-sprayed pan or oil on an open fire or in the oven. The protease inhibitors in the seeds get deactivated after fifteen to twenty minutes of cooking. This, in turn, makes the seeds more digestible than normal. The cover/coating of the seeds is edible, too, and just like pumpkin seeds, it contains a lot of insoluble fiber. The seeds like are like mesquite pods, which means they can be dried and then ground into flour. The roots are full of starch and can be mashed, and then the starch can be leached in water. The cellulose present in the root is bitter. Remove the cellulose from the water if you want to reduce the bitterness. The root water can be fermented to make alcoholic beverages. The plant can also prove to be commercially viable in arid and semi-arid lands, especially where there is ample need for starch, protein, and oil. If you find the taste of this plant too bitter, it is recommended to avoid it altogether.

Uses

The hollow, dried gourd was used to make a musical instrument that was used for various rituals, which may precede 10,000 years. The dried root can be used as an emetic. The root can be used to make a decoction that can be used to treat sexually transmitted diseases. The root of the plant often looks a bit 'humanoid.' This is why, according to the Doctrine of Signatures, Native Americans would dig up the root and cut the section, which looks like a human body part. This section was then prepared in a special way to treat the real body part similar to the root. Crushed leaves and stems were used as a poultice for infections and various sores.

In modern medicine, buffalo gourd is often used as a laxative. Certain holistic practitioners still follow traditional methods of usage. A lot of research is necessary to prove the health and medical benefits of this plant.

The saponins present in the roots of the plant can be mashed and mixed with water. This often leads to the formation of suds which can be used to clean various things in emergencies. This liquid also has antimicrobial properties.

Caution

Although the plant is closely related to squashes, it can prove to be toxic. Only consume prepared seeds and avoid other parts.

Sage

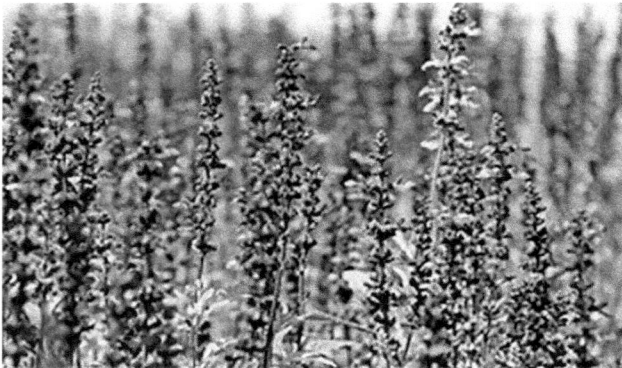

Asteraceae (Artemisia tridentate Nutt.)

Identification

It is a fragrant, grayish shrub that grows up to 7'. The leaves are shaped like wedges and have lobes. They taper at the base but are broad at the tip. The plant produces brownish-yellowish flowers which grow in narrow clusters. The plant generally blooms between the period of July to October. The seed is hairy. The plant is also known as a sagebrush.

Habitat

It is one of the most popular dry-area, a shrub in Washington, Wyoming, Montana, New Mexico, Texas, Idaho, California, Colorado, Oregon, and various other places in the West.

Edible

The seeds, whether dried or raw, can be grounded into the floor or can be eaten from hand. Seeds can also be added to liqueurs to add flavor and fragrance to them.

Harvest

Harvest the seeds upon the maturation of the plant. The leaves can be harvested throughout the lifecycle of the plant.

Uses

It is a potent warrior plant that was used extensively for sweeping and smudging to get rid of the evil spirits and bad airs. A tea made with the leaves can be used to ease childbirth, treat infections, and wash sore eyes. The soaked leaves can also be used as a poultice over wounds. The tea was used to treat stomach problems and pain. The limbs are often added to baths. The infusion made with the leaves can also be used to treat coughs, colds, throat infections, and bronchitis. The infusion or decoction can be used externally as a wash for pimples, sores, cuts, etc. The decoction is aromatic and can be inhaled to treat headaches and respiratory problems. The decoction is antirheumatic and antidiarrheal. The infusion was also used as a remedy against constipation and other digestive ailments.

In modern times Native Americans still use the herb for a variety of ritualistic purposes, including sweeping, smudging, disinfecting, and as a sweat lodge. The oil of the A. tridentate variety is potent against gram-positive bacteria.

Notes
This herb can be added to the hot tub or bath for a relaxing and cleansing bath. It is often the only source of firewood in deserts.

Prickly Pear
Cactaceae (Opuntia spp.)

Identification
It generally grows in arid and desert lands. The plant has large oval pads with various-sized thorny leaves. The flowers are yellow. The fruits are varied and are generally white, red, purple, or in between.

Habitat

They are easily found from coast to coast in badlands, sandy areas, deserts, etc. They are often found in Wyoming, eastern Colorado, Utah, and other dry areas of other states.

Harvest

Various parts of the plant can be harvested upon maturation.

Edible

The pads are often mistaken for leaves, but the thorns are the real leaves that have been modified over the years to conserve water. The pads are edible. Most of the edible species have flat joints connecting the pads. The flower buds and flowers are edible and are roasted and eaten. Species that have fat pads can be roasted and eaten. It is recommended to use fresh pads. The fire burns off the thorns and cooks the pads thoroughly. Once cooked, let the pads cool and then peel the skin to eat the core flesh. You can also slice the core and stir-fry it. Flowers of most of the species are edible, and Native Americans often consume them, but do not try unless you are well aware of the toxicity of the plant. The fruit becomes red on ripening. It is tasty, and it can be made into jelly as well. It has prickly hair, so be careful while eating. The pads can be mixed with yeast, water, and sugar and fermented to make an alcoholic drink. The raw, green fruit can be cooked and eaten as well.

Uses

The flowers are astringent and can be crushed to make a poultice over wounds. The tea made using the flowers are used to treat various stomach ailments such as IBS or irritable bowel syndrome and

311

diarrhea. Roast the leaf pads on an open fire. This will burn off the thorns. Slice the pads in half and use the moist side as a poultice on infections, wounds, stings, and bites. This provides cleansing and sealing effects on the wounds. The thorn-less pads can be cooked, sliced, and applied as a poultice on breasts to increase milk. The O. polyacantha variety is used to make an infusion that is traditionally used to treat diarrhea.

In modern times, people from the American Southwest and Mexico still use the plant for its traditional uses. The flowers are still used as a remedy for enlarged prostates. The core of the pad is a surfactant, chemotactic attractant, etc. and it draws serum from the wound, which cleans and seals the wound. The fruit can be sliced, peeled, and eaten with some cayenne pepper. The juice made from the fruit is hypoglycemic and has anti-inflammatory properties.

Rabbitbrush, Brushbar

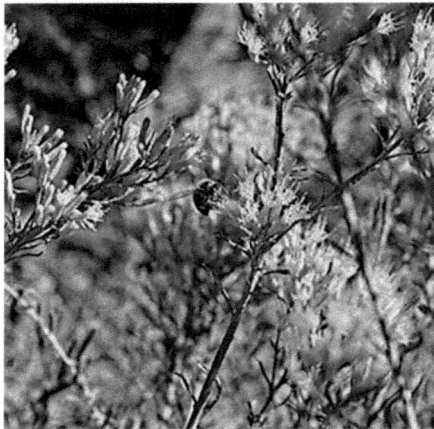

Asteraceae (Ericameria nauseosa [Pall ex Pursh] GL Nesom & GI Baird)

Identification

The plant is densely branched, erect shrub, which grows up to 10' tall. The leaves are narrow and elongated. The flowers are yellow and grow in heads. The fruits are achenes tufted that have white hair. There are many different species available throughout the nation. It is also known as rabbitbrush.

Habitat

They are found in montane and dry areas. They are easily found in Washington State, Montana, and in British Columbia. Dry, lower montane areas and desert, from Montana. The plant is also found in West Texas, the Osoyoos area of the southern Okanagan valley, and in southeastern California. It prefers gravelly, sandy, alkali, or dry soil. It is generally found at low elevations but can also be seen at higher elevations.

Harvest

Various parts of the plant can be harvested upon maturation.

Edible

The latex of the root and the inner bark are both used as chewing gum. While there is no record of toxicity of the plant, it is better to avoid its bitter taste.

Uses

The blossoms were used to make yellow dyes, while the stems were used to make baskets by the Native Americans from the southwest. A decoction made with the roots is used to treat fevers, colds, coughs, etc. The root decoction can be used to relieve menstrual cramps. The leaves are crushed and infused to make remedies for headaches and the crushed leaves can also be used to relieve dental pain. The tea made using the leaves of the plant can be used to treat stomach problems. The tea has laxative properties.

Yucca

Agavaceae (Yucca spp.: Y. filamentosa L.; Y. glauca Nutt.; Y. baccata Torr.)

Identification

It is medium to large-sized, robust perennial. It has an ever-growing rootstock which grows in colonies and clumps. The leaves are like a sword and come out from the basal rosettes. They are fibrous, tough, green, long, and waxy. The flowers can be cream-colored or white and are shaped either like a bowl or a bell. They bloom on woody, tall spikes that go beyond the leaves. The plant blooms from May to July. It is also known as Adam's needle, Joshua tree, or Spanish bayonet.

Habitat

It is mostly found in high plains, upland prairies, sandy blowouts, deserts, and California coastal hillsides.

Harvest

The flowers can be harvested from May. The leaves and roots can be harvested upon maturation.

Edible

The while flowers can be consumed by adding them to omelets and frittatas. You can also use the flowers as a garnish or add them to salads. The fruits of almost all the species are edible, but some are more edible than others. For instance, the Y. baccata variety has large and succulent fruits that taste bland but are full of flavonoids.

Uses

According to various folklore and similar claims, the root decoction is supposed to be highly beneficial for hair and can even regrow it. The infusion made with crushed roots can be used as a remedy for headaches. The root of Yucca is a surfactant, i.e., it is a wetting agent, which means it can pop the cell membranes of microbes, which makes it a great soap. The decoction of Yucca roots is still used to kill lice and to wash hair. The decoction can be ingested internally to treat arthritis, but more study is required. The roots of the Y. filamentosa variety contains steroid saponins, which can be used to make a decoction to treat liver and gallbladder problems. The smashed leaves can be used to stop vomiting, while the infusion of the roots can be used as a laxative. The root is considered to be a male warrior plant which is used in various smudging rituals. These rituals are done to get rid of bad spirits and bad airs from the body. The roots of the Y. baccata variety was used to soothe the process and pain of childbirth.

In modern medicine, the plant still finds multiple uses. For instance, in Europe, the leaves are dried and ground and used for various purposes. The extracts of leaves and roots are still used to treat gallbladder and liver problems. Taking too much steroid saponin can lead to nausea and other stomach problems.

The saponin present in the plant can kill lyse and generate suds that are still used as a ritualistic shampoo.

Notes

The flower shoots i.e., the stalks, are dried and uses as arrows by Native Americans. They are also used as Indian matches.

Yaupon

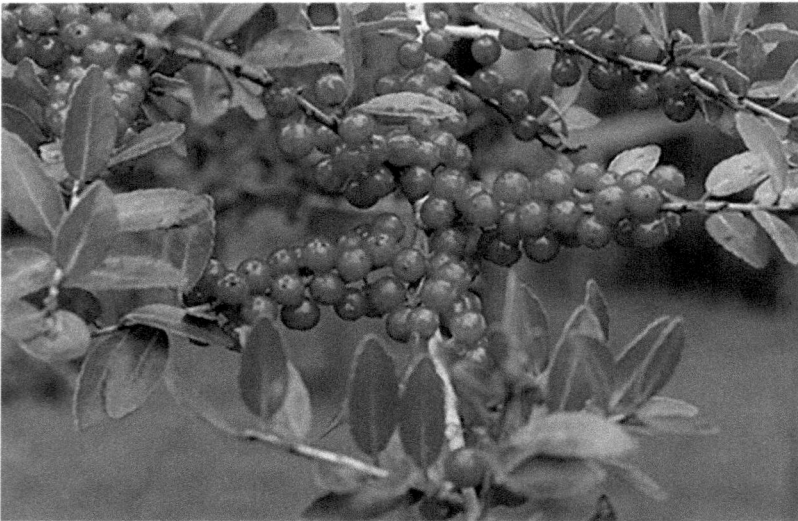

Aquifoliaceae (Ilex vomitoria Ait.)

Identification

It is a shrub-like plant with alternating, oval, and glossy green leaves. The margins have round teeth and the leaves are generally 1" wide. The plant is also known as yaupon holly.

Habitat

It is commonly found in Texas and similar places and it can also be found in North Carolina. It is almost a desert plant.

Edible

The berries are toxic, but the leaves can be roasted to make tea. Roast the young leaves at 200 F until they turn brown. Crush the eaves and put a teaspoon of them in hot water. Cool the beverage and drink.

Uses

Many different First People nations used the fruits and leaves for ritual healings. The roasted leaves were used to make a decoction used as an emetic and to purge the internal systems. The decoction was supposed to dispel nightmares and it can also cure restlessness and sleep-talking. It is supposed to have hallucinogenic properties.

The roasted leaves can be steeped in water to make tea, which is stimulant and diuretic. Native Americans use stronger teas and infusions for purification rituals, where they purify the body with the help of vomiting. The tea is stimulating because it contains a lot of caffeine. Yaupon is perhaps the only plant native to the United States of America, which contains caffeine in its leaves naturally.

Caution

The berries are toxic.

Note: The berries and leaves are used to make dyes. The ripe berries are red and are used to make red dye. The dye can be used to dye wool and other similar material. To make gray, leaves are crushed and mixed with either copper or iron.

Agave

Agavaceae (Agave spp.: A. americana L.)

Identification

It is a desert plant that grows up to 10'. It has long, grayish-green, succulent leaves that look like swords and the flowers bloom on the central fruiting spike. The plant is also called an American century plant.

Habitat

It is generally found in the arid areas of Arizona, California, Mexico, and Nevada. It can also be found in South and Central America.

Harvest

The roots can be harvested upon maturation.

Edible

The roots of the American century plant can be cooked in a pit. These cooked roots are then crushed and fermented. The young leaves can be roasted and then kept away for future use. The young buds, fruit heads, and flower stalks, all are edible and are roasted before consuming. Agave is used to make vino mescal, pulque, and tequila. To make mescal, the 'leaves' are chopped from the middle of the plant, and the liquid is allowed to drip into the hold. A farmer then sucks out the watery sap in the gourd. This sap is then kept away for fermentation for around a week and is served fresh. This water is potable drinking water. It is a wildly cultivated and used plant in the Hispanic community. The popularity of tequila has made this plant popular as well.

The tender inner core of the middle leaves is often cooked and consumed.

Uses

Agave water, i.e., sap/juice, is considered to be a diuretic and anti-inflammatory. Fresh juice can increase perspiration and metabolism. In modern medicine, the leaf waste is collected, concentrated, and used as the raw material for hecogenin, a steroid drug.

The roots of agave contain saponins which produce suds and are thus used to manufacture soap. The fiber from the leaves is coarse and is often used to make fiber and ropes. The sap is still used as a laxative and a demulcent. The sap can be used for sealing as well as treating wounds.

Gumweed

Asteraceae (Grindelia camporum Green; G. integrifolia DC.; G. nana Nutt.)

Identification

All the species of this plant are almost similar, and all of them are erect perennials or biennials. The leaves are alternate, light green, serrated (can also be smooth). The stem is clasping and is dotted with resin. The flowers are generally yellow or orangish-yellow and look like dandelions. The bracts of the flowers are sticky and viscous, which is why the plant is known as Gumweed.

Habitat

The G. camporum variety is found in California, British Columbia, Sonora Desert, and other similar places while the G. integrifolia variety is found in salt marshes, open coastlines, etc. The G. nana variety is generally found in Idaho.

Not Edible

Uses

The plant was often used to treat respiratory infections in the past. The Native Americans used the parts of the plant to make decoctions for multiple uses. It was used topically to treat wounds, poison oak, poison ivy, dermatitis, and boils. The sap from flowers and leaves was often used on sores.

In modern medicine, it is used to treat cough and bronchitis. The drug is supposed to have antifungal, antimicrobial, and anti-inflammatory properties. The dried aerial parts are used to make tinctures and teas.

Caution

Large doses can be toxic and can lead to gastric problems.

Mormon Tea

Ephedraceae (Ephedra Viridis Coville; E. Sinica)

Identification

There are many different joint fir species. The E. virdis variety looks like it has no leaves, is yellowish-green, twiggy, and has multiple joints. The plant is short and has small leaf scales. Upon maturation, in fall, it produces double seeded cones. It looks leggy as it generally does not have a lot of leaves. It is also known as ma huang, joint fir, or ephedra.

Habitat

Multiple species are found on sandy, rocky, or dry soil. These are found mainly in desert-areas in the states of Arizona, Utah, New Mexico, Nevada, Colorado, California, Oregon, Nevada, etc.

Harvest

The seeds can be harvested upon maturation. The aerial parts can be harvested when the plant is young.

Edible

The roasted seeds were used to make infusions by the Native Americans. The roasted and ground seeds were mixed with wheat or cornflour to make mush.

Uses

Mormon tea or E. Viridis was used as a laxative or a tonic to treat colds, anemia, ulcers, diarrhea, and backache. It was also used to improve the health of the bladder and the kidneys. The infusion or the decoction was used as a blood purifier or a cleansing tonic. The dried and powdered stems were used topically on sores and wounds. The powder was mixed with water to make a paste that was applied to burns by the Native Americans. The First People used it to stimulate menstruation. The roasted seeds were used to make a tea-like beverage.

In modern times the E. Sinica variety is used extensively for its medicinal benefits. For instance, in China, the dried stems are ground to make a powder that is used to treat bronchitis, coughs, congestion, bronchial asthma, obesity, and hay fever. It is also used to suppress appetite and to enhance metabolism. American ephedra is available over the counter in the form of capsules or tea and has almost no vasoactive effects.

Caution

E. Sinica is a CNS (central nervous system) and cardiovascular stimulant. It is generally dangerous for people who have heart diseases, high blood pressure, or tachycardia. It is regulated federally and should not be used by pregnant or new mothers. It also interacts with a lot of drugs, which is why its import and use are restricted in multiple countries. Abusing the drug may lead to deaths.

Jojoba

Simmodsiaceae (Simmondsia Chinensis [Link], Schneid.)

Identification

It is an evergreen, dioecious shrub, which means it is a separate sexed plant. It has many branches and bluish-green leaves that are paired and oblong. Both the male and female flowers are small. The male flower is yellow while the female is pale-green. The fruit capsule bears one to three seeds.

Habitat

It is found in the Southwest Desert and the Sonora Desert. It is also found in Mexico. It is cultivated as a crop in the Southwest to extract liquid wax.

Harvest

The seeds are harvested upon maturation.

Edible

The seeds are ground to make percolations or decoctions to make beverages. The kernel of the seed is waxy, and it can be baked or boiled and consumed. It can also be blended and added to the cake mix. The nuts can be shelled and consumed and the nut kernels are used to make nut butter.

Uses

The Southwestern Native Americans crushed the dry nuts to make a poultice for sores and wounds. The powder made from the fruit was ingested internally for cathartic reasons. This powder was also used topically to treat psoriasis and acne. The green, raw seeds of jojoba were chewed on to treat sore throats.

In modern medicine, the oil made from jojoba is used for a variety of skincare products. It is used as a carrier oil. The oil contains extracts that prevent oxidation. According to certain studies, the oil also has the potential to lower cholesterol; however, extra studies are needed.

Notes

It is a widespread plant in the Southwest and is cultivated there as a crop. The oil extracted from the seeds can be used for a variety of cosmetic purposes.

Chaparral

Zygophyllaceae (Larrea tridentata [Sessé & Moc. ex DC.], Coville)

Identification

It is an aromatic and resinous shrub that is generally 6' tall. It has reddish-brown bark around the base, which becomes almost white towards the top. The branches and limbs are light-colored as well. The leaves are yellowish-green, tiny, and look and feel like leather. The flowers, too, are yellow and small and grow into hairy seed-bearing pods upon maturation. The plant is also known as creosote bush.

Habitat

It is generally found in deserts, especially in Mexico Southwestern United States.

Not Edible

Toxic

Uses

The Native Americans used the decoction made with the evergreen leaves of the plant to treat various stomach problems such as diarrhea. The chewed plant is used to make a poultice that can be applied over spider bites, insect bites, and snakebites. The leaf infusion can be used as a wash to increase milk flow. The heated twigs release a sap, which was packed in cavities to cure toothache. The poultice made from leaves was applied to various skin problems, wounds, and chest to prevent chest complaints.

Native Americans also used the plant as a treatment for sexually transmitted diseases, rheumatic diseases, cancer (especially leukemia), and urinary tract infections. The leaves were used to make tea, which was used as a pulmonary antiseptic and as an expectorant.

Chaparral was used extensively to treat many different conditions, including colds, influenza, fever, gas, sinusitis, anemia, arthritis, premenstrual syndrome, fungal infections, autoimmune diseases, etc. until recently. It is still considered to be a diuretic, analgesic, antidiarrheal, and emetic. The aerial parts are washed, dried, and ground to make a powder that can be used for multiple purposes.

Caution

Now the medical and commercial value of this plant is under question because its potential toxicity which affects the liver and can lead to acute or subacute hepatitis. Chaparral contains NDGA or nordihydroguaiaretic acid, which is a strong antioxidant that can promote cancer and inhibit it. Due to these two factors, viz. liver issues and cancer-causing potential, the plant is now falling out of use, and people are looking for new, better, and safer options instead. It is advised to avoid consuming the plant in the form of teas, capsules, loose leaves, and in the form of bulk herbal products as it can prove to be harmful to the kidneys and the heart.

Some holistic health-care practitioners still use and prescribe the herb, but it is better to check with a licensed professional first. Do not use if you are not sure of the results.

Notes

One of the main reasons why chaparral grows so well and in abundance is thanks to its survival method. The plant contains high amounts of a very toxic substance released and produced by its roots. This prevents other plants from growing near it. When it rains, the toxins are washed away, allowing other plants to grow around it, but as soon as the water drains away, the toxin is released again, effectively killing all the other plants. This is an important ability in the desert because it allows chaparral to survive without having to compete with other plants for the already scarce resources and nutrients.

Chapter 6

Herbs and Plants of the West Coast

Here is a list of some of the most commonly found medicinal plants, herbs, and trees of the West Coast.

Devil's Club

Aralioideae (Oplopanax horridus Sm. Torr. & Gray ex Miq)

Identification

It is a perennial shrub that grows up to 10' tall. It is crooked, spreads densely, and has sharp thorns. The wood has a sweet aroma and the leaves are huge and look like maple leaves. The flower head looks like a club and the flowers are generally white while the berries are flattened and bright red.

Habitat

It is generally found along coastlines and coastal mountains. It is found on stream banks, near seepage sites, moist forested areas, and avalanche tracks. It generally grows in low altitude but may also grow in higher altitudes.

Not Edible

Uses

The plant is related to ginseng, and its berries, roots, and greenish bark are used for various medical purposes. It is considered to be one of the most important medicinal plants of the area. The First People still use the herb as a medicine and in various rituals.

The berries are crushed and rubbed in the hair to make it shiny and to kill lice. The inner bark of the plant can be chewed upon raw or can be consumed with hot water for emetic and purgative purposes. The inner bark can be used to make decoctions or infusions to treat arthritis, bowel and stomach cramps, ulcers, and various other unspecified problems of the digestive system. The leaves, roots, and stems are often added to sweat lodges and baths as a remedy against arthritis. The shredded and cooked root bark can be used as a poultice for a variety of skin problems. The decoction of the stem can be used to bring down a fever.

The tea from the inner bark can be used to treat diabetes. To cure headaches, the dried root was mixed with tobacco and smoked. An infusion made with the stem of the plant is used as a tonic and a blood purifier. Oil and stem ashes were used topically for many different skin issues. It was also used as an abortifacient traditionally; however, the use has been disproved now.

Native Americans still practice the traditional uses of this plant. According to certain German studies, it was found that this plant has analgesic and anti-inflammatory properties. Certain animal studies prove that the extracts of the roots can be used to reduce heart rate and blood pressure.

Western Red Cedar

Cupressaceae (Thuja plicata D. Don.)

Identification

It is an aromatic evergreen tree that can grow up to 230' tall. It has many branches with flattened needles. It produces seed crops every three years. The tree becomes mature at around the age of twenty.

Habitat

It is found in moist areas with deep and rich soil. It grows around Vancouver Island, the Windward side of the Cascades, etc.

Harvest

The bark can be harvested once hard.

Edible

T. plicata is mostly used to make planks and cooking boxes that are used for cooking and flavor salmon. The inner bark can be consumed as a survival food; however, it should only be used as a last resort as you are more likely to find better and safer options around.

Uses

The red cedar is a male warrior plant that is used by the Native Americans for smudging, sweeping, and steam-bath rituals to purify the mind and the body and to get read of unhealthy conditions and evil spirits.

The tribes from the Northwest use the wood to make cedar boxes that are used for storage and cooking both. Europeans use the wood to line chests as it can repel insects, and it smells good. The dried and powdered leaves are used to make a decoction, which is used topically to treat injuries, sores, painful joints, and wounds. The infusion made with leaves can also be used to treat colds and coughs. The decoction made with the bark was used to induce menstruation and thus is said to have abortifacient properties. The new and tender leaf buds are supposed to be good for lung problems. The boughs and leaves can be used to make a decoction to treat arthritis.

In modern homeopathic medicine, practitioners prefer T. occidentalis to T. plicata. It is used to treat poor digestion, rheumatism, skin problems, and depression.

Caution

As the plant contains thujone, it is advised not to use this drug without proper professional supervision and consultation. Improper use may lead to the development of a variety of problems.

Juniper

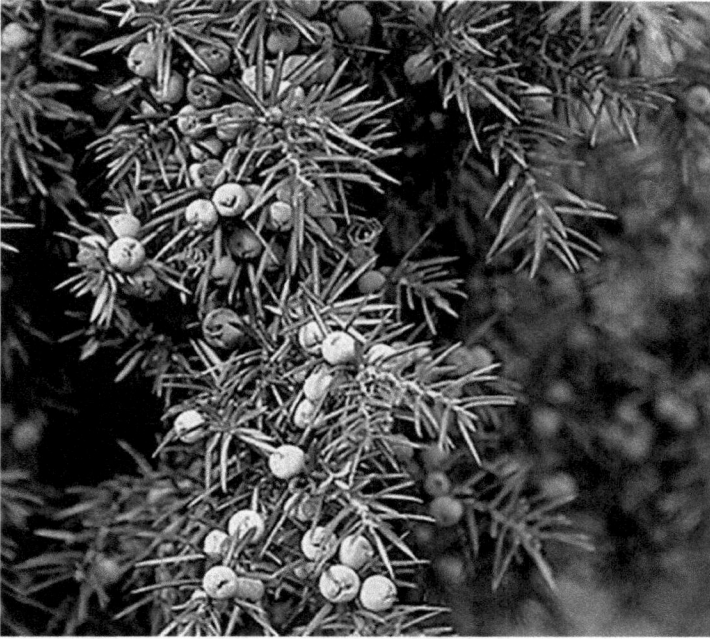

Cupressaceae (Juniperus communis L.; Juniperus osteosperma [Torr. Little)

Identification

It can either be a low-lying shrub or an evergreen tree. It often grows in colonies. The leaves are stiff, evergreen, pointy, slightly flat, and light green. The buds are covered with needles and the berries are blue and tangy. The male flowers have numerous stamens arranged in three whorls and look like catkin. The female flowers are green and oval. The fruits, upon maturation, become blue, aromatic, edible. They generally have one or more seeds.

Habitat

The J. communis variety is found throughout the nation, while the J. osteosperma variety is generally found Wyoming and the southwest.

Harvest

The berries can be harvested once ripe. Other parts can be harvested throughout the life cycle.

Edible

The dried berries are used to flavor fowl and game. You can also put the berries in a pepper mill to grind them into stews, bean soup, goat, lamb, duck, venison, and turkey. The berries can also be used to make tea. Juniper berries are used to flavor vodka, gin, aquavit, and schnapps. You can also add the berries to marinades. Do not use too many berries as they can prove to be toxic (just like salt and pepper). Use the berries like a spice.

Uses

The essential oil (diluted) can be used to cleanse deeper skin tissues. The extracts have been used to treat dysmenorrhea, PMS, and to promote menstruation. Some practitioners also add needles and bark to the tea made with berries. The berry has diuretic, antiseptic, and digestive properties. It can be used as a tonic. It is great for the problems of the urinary tract and the gallbladder. It should not be used if the person has kidney issues.

According to modern medicine, the extracts can be used to treat dyspepsia. The extract of the berries has diuretic properties. The extracts can be used to treat dropsy, heart diseases, and high blood pressure and it is used to treat gout and arthritis in Europe. Research is going on to study the anticancer, anti-diabetes, and anti-inflammatory properties of the extracts.

Caution

Use juniper carefully and sparingly as it can lead to allergies. A pregnant woman should avoid using the plant altogether as it may lead to uterine contractions. It can also increase menstrual bleeding.

Do not use juniper if you have kidney diseases, kidney infection, or have symptoms of a kidney problem. Do not use caustic and concentrated essential oil without consulting a licensed holistic medical professional.

Sweet Cicely

Apiaceae (Myrrhis Odorata L. Scop.)

Identification

This plant looks like hemlock but is smaller, growing up to 3' tall. The crushed roots smell like anise seeds and the leaves are bright green and shiny, while the flowers are small, white, and in umbels. It is also known as wild anise and has a sweet anise aroma and taste. The flowers bloom in early summer or late spring, are shaped like a pyramid and are generally brownish-black. The leaves taste like anise and smell like lovage.

Habitat

It is generally found throughout the United States of America except on high mountains and extreme deserts. It is a forest dweller. It prefers good soil and shade.

Harvest

The roots and leaves are edible and can be harvest around spring. Be careful! The plant looks like a poison hemlock, and it is easy to confuse between them.

Edible

Both the root and leaves are edible but should be harvested with the utmost care as the plant looks like poison hemlock. Do not harvest if you are confused. The root is used as a spice in baked goods, cooked greens, etc. It can be used as an anise substitute. The leaves are often used in salads. The cooked root can be pickled, added to soups, salads, and can be consumed cold too.

Uses

Traditionally it is used as an expectorant and a blood purifier for hundreds of years. It was also used to treat breathing problems and asthma.

In modern times the tea made using the roots is used as a decongestant, an expectorant, and as a digestive aid. The root is still thought to be effective against anemia thanks to the high iron content present in the roots. The cooked root acts as a carminative.

Sweet Clover

Fabaceae (Melilotus officinalis L. Pall.)

Identification

It is a small, heavily branched plant with yellow flowers. The leaves are finely toothed and alternate. They are trifoliate i.e.; they have three petioles. The small, yellow flowers bloom profusely on stemmed racemes. The fruit has a thorny tip; it is smooth, obtuse, and brownish-black. It generally has one seed per pod. The plant is also known as yellow sweet clover.

Habitat

It is generally found in the east of the Mississippi and prairie states. It can also be found on mountain meadows. It is available throughout the United States of America.

Harvest

The root and flowers can be harvested upon maturation.

Not Edible

Sweet clover contains coumarins, which are anticoagulants and act as blood thinners. This has killed cattle in the past. Do not eat.

Uses

The roots and flowers were used by Native Americans to make an infusion, which was used as a wash to treat sunburn and pimples. The aerial parts have been used in the past to make cold infusions by Ramah Navajo to treat colds.

The dried flowers were smudged on the house to bring in good spirits.

In modern medicine, the stems, flowers, and leaves have been used to procure extracts, which can be used to treat edema, blunt injuries, varicose veins, wounds, and hemorrhoids. It is supposed to have anti-inflammatory properties. It can improve lymphatic and venous performance.

Caution

The plant contains various flavonoids, volatile oils, coumarins, and saponins, so use strictly under the medical supervision of a licensed professional.

Western Hemlock

Pinaceae (Tsuga heterophylla [Raf.] Sarg.)

Identification

It is a tall evergreen plant that can grow up to 150' tall. It has a conical, narrow crown with drooping branches. The needles are flexible, flat, and rounded at the tip. It has brownish-yellow, slender twigs with fine hair that is rough to touch. The cones are long, elliptical, brown, and do not have a stalk. They generally hang at the end of the twig. The seeds are long-winged and paired.

Habitat

It is generally found in southern Alaska and California and is also found in Montana and Idaho. It prefers moist and acidic soils and likes lower slopes and low flats.

Harvest

The bark can be harvested upon maturation.

Edible

The inner bark was used to make bread by the Native Americans living on the coast.

Uses

The outer bark was used to make a decoction, which was used as a wash to treat burns and wounds. The inner bark was infused and scrapped to treat acute infections, including colds, flu, etc. The resin and oil from hemlock are used externally to get relief from rheumatic joints, and arthritis. The needles are used to make tea, which is high in vitamin C. This tea can help you prevent scurvy.

In modern times the teas and decoctions are still used by the First People for a variety of purposes. The hemlock boughs are used to harvest herring eggs by First People. Modern medicine rarely uses hemlock for its medicinal properties.

Caution

The tea made from the needles is used to treat flu and colds, but it can be toxic if taken in large amounts.

Notes

Hemlock is great pulpwood is used to make cellophane paper, plastics, and rayon. Native Americans use it to make paddles, fishing lures, and boats.

Buckthorn

Rhamnaceae (Rhamnus cathartica L.; R. purshiana [DC.] Cooper)

Identification

It is a medium-sized bush or a small tree that may grow up to 20' tall. It has many branches and densely foliated. While the name suggests otherwise, the plant is completely sans thorns. Upon maturation, the bark turns grayish-brown with grayish-white lenticels. The leaves are hairy, thin, elliptical, and fully margined. The greenish-white flowers grow in abundance on the axillary cymes. They are tiny and have five petals. The ripe fruit is generally reddish-purple to purplish-black and has two or more seeds. The R. purshiana variety is taller and has larger leaves.

Habitat

R. cathartica is generally found in dune-lands around Lake Michigan. R. purshiana is found at the foothills of Idaho, British Columbia, Montana, Washington, and Oregon.

Not Edible

Uses

Before World War II, Cascara pills were available over the counter as a laxative. Native Americans used the infusions made from the bark for its laxative, purgative, and worm-killing properties. An infusion made with the fruit and the twigs were used as an emetic. To reduce the harshness of the bark, it can be cured for a year or so.

Even in the modern days, the extract of the bark of R. purshiana is considered to be a potent laxative. It is used to treat constipation. The result/response of this drug may last up to eight hours.

Caution

Never use this drug to clear intestinal obstructions. The infusion of the bark is considered to be a cleansing tonic, but using it for a long time can prove to be carcinogenic. It is recommended to use this drug only under the guidance of a licensed holistic or any other form of a medical professional.

American Yew

Rhamnaceae (Taxus brevifolia Nutt.)

Identification

It is an evergreen shrub that grows up to 50' tall. The bark is reddish-purple, drooping, and papery. The leaves are flat and like needles and grow in opposite rows. The flowers are shaped like small cones. The fruit is small, berrylike, scarlet, and have a fleshy cup around the seed.

Habitat

It is generally found in Oregon, Northern California, Washington, Montana, Idaho, Alberta, and British Columbia. It prefers shady and moist sites.

Edible

The Mendocino and Karok tribes consumed the ripe and red fruit. All the other parts of the plant are considered to be toxic and should not be consumed. It is recommended to avoid the food as well.

Uses

The wet needles of T. brevifolia, i.e., American yew was used by Native Americans as a poultice on wounds. The needles were considered to be a strong and powerful tonic, a panacea, and used for a variety of purposes including treating injuries and reducing pain. The decoctions made using the bark were used to cure stomachache. It was first used by the Native Americans to treat cancer.

In modern times American yew is used to make taxine or paclitaxel. It is a toxic drug the halts the process of cell multiplication and is useful in treating cancer. It is often used to treat the cancer of cervix, leukemia, breast, and ovary. More and more clinical trials are necessary.

Caution

Both the species can be quite harmful and may induce abortion. All parts of the plant are toxic and should not be consumed unless advised by a licensed holistic professional.

Notes

Both species have cancer-fighting properties. It takes around 9000 kg dried bark or 3000 trees (T. brevifolia) to make just one kg of Taxol. This rate of extraction will destroy all the wild yew trees in the United States of America. To counter this nowadays, Taxol is produced by cloning cells in gigantic bioreactor tanks. Researchers are nowadays working on producing pinene from pine trees.

Conclusion

The rise of various diseases and disorders have scared people all around the world. Modern medicine is helpful, but it has its problems, the foremost being its multitude of side-effects and steep rates. It is no wonder that a lot of people have once again started moving towards ancient practices and herbal medicine.

Herbal and medicinal plants grow throughout the world. Many different and highly useful species grow in the United States of America. Some of them are well-known, while others are not. These herbs and plants hold the secret to a long, healthy, and fit life. You just need to learn how to unlock them. These herbs can surely make our lives full of wellness and health.

It should not come as a surprise then that foraging is rapidly gaining popularity all over the world, especially in the United States of America. It is not only a hobby anymore; it has become a life choice that is healthy, helpful, and sustainable if performed properly. It is necessary to learn how to identify and forage wild plants as it can help you in a variety of ways. It needs to be a continuous journey. You should passionately seek more and more plants and information related to them.

While this book does contain a lot of data related to some of the most common (and certain uncommon) plants, it is still incomplete. In fact, no book can contain a detailed list of all the medicinal plants because Mother Nature has blessed these plants with an open heart. This book will help you identify many different plants and will also inform you about their health benefits, but instead of stopping here, look for even more plants.

Detailed data on the basics of foraging, common herbs, storage, and preservation will not only help you identify the plants but will also help you to collect and store them. While the book is centered on North America, many of the plants can be found at other places too. Thus, this book will help you to harness the gifts of Mother Nature without harming her.

Identifying, gathering, and using wild medicinal plants is a beautiful experience. It allows you to form a better, greater connection with Mother Nature. You become one with her when you experience the gentle healing action of leaves, roots, flowers, fruits, and various other parts of the plants. It is not just a medical experience; it is a spiritual awakening as well. It is a chance to go back to the roots.

Always remember, herbalism and foraging should be done with the utmost respect. There are enough herbs in nature for everyone's need, but not for everyone's greed. Do not destroy a plant or a species for your greed. Wanton foraging should be avoided. This book contains tips regarding wanton foraging and how to avoid it, which will help you forage sustainably.

While modern medicines and drugs are often avoided for their side-effects, wild plants and herbs can have side-effects too. Certain herbs are extremely potent, and misusing or abusing them can lead to various severe problems. It is recommended to contact a proper, licensed health professional or a doctor before using any herb, plant, or extract.

Foraging can be a remarkable experience if you try to connect with nature. Good luck!

References

Adamant, A. (2018, November 9). 16 Medicinal Trees for Your
    Herbal Medicine Chest. Practical Self Reliance website:
    https://practicalselfreliance.com/medicinal-trees/

Burns, J. (2018, August 1). Foraging for Food and Herbs — ROISH
    Herbal Apothecary & Nutritional Wellness | Herbal
    Apothecary & Nutritional Wellness. ROISH Herbal
    Apothecary & Nutritional Wellness website:
    https://www.roishherbalapothecary.com/the-
    articles/2018/4/26/template-d36kc

Codekas, C. (2019, April 3). What to Forage in Spring: 20 Edible
    and Medicinal Plants and Fungi Grow Forage Cook Ferment
    website: https://www.growforagecookferment.com/what-to-
    forage-in-spring/

Erich. (2019, July 29). A Guide to Foraging for Medicinal Plants.
    Hobby Farms website: https://www.hobbyfarms.com/a-
    guide-to-foraging-for-medicinal-plants/

Foraging For Wild Edibles and Medicinals Archives. (n.d.).
    Chestnut School of Herbal Medicine website:

https://chestnutherbs.com/category/foraging-for-wild-edibles-and-medicinals/

Foraging for Wild Edibles and Medicine with Planty Kim | Abundance Healing Arts. (n.d.). https://abundancehealingarts.com/herbalism-wild-foods/

Free Food and Medicine (Part 1): Make Foraging for Edible and Medicinal Plants and Mushrooms Part of Your Every Day Wilderness Experience. (n.d.). wms.org website: https://wms.org/magazine/1241/Free_Food_and_Medicine

Meuninck, J. (2016). Medicinal plants of North America : a field guide. Guilford, Connecticut: Falconguides.

Middleton, J. (1984). Proceedings of the Symposium on the Role of Biology in Development, Dar es Salaam, September 1983. Dar Es Salaam: Published By The Faculty Of Science, University Of Dar Es Salaam In Collaboration With The Tanzania National Scientific Research Council.

Opsomer, L. (2019, March 6). Foraging in North America. Adventure Publications website: http://blog.adventurepublications.net/2019/03/foraging-in-north-america/

FORAGING

FOR BEGINNERS

*Identifying Fruits, Nuts
and Seeds in North America*

MONA GREENY

Introduction

Humans used to be much more self-sufficient way back in the day. From discovering fire to agriculture and trade, we have evolved into superior beings, or have we? With the invention of the wheel, we stopped walking. With agriculture and livestock farming, we stopped hunting and growing food and with the emergence of processed food and delivery, we stopped cooking at home. We can see a pattern here that tells us that as we progress with science and technology, we are moving further from where we came from as human beings. Today, an average person cannot cook, clean, or do basic tasks without a professional involved, be it a chef at their favorite restaurant, a maid to clean their house, or an electrician to change a light bulb. As we expand our abilities in terms of technology and business development, we are slowly becoming distant from basic skills that generations before us were accustomed to. One of the most important skills that made humans who were are today was foraging. By definition, foraging is simply the acquisition of food and supplies from the wild. It has been done by our ancestors for thousands of years, and long before farming and agriculture were ever a thing.

Since the commercialization of food production, humans have little or no knowledge of how food is grown, let alone alternative options easily available in the wild. This is because we have changed our ways and are completely reliant on systemized economies to survive. The last decade has seen a series of events that are changing the way people are living. A lot of people are downsizing to meet expenses while others are following the environmental initiative. Whatever it is, people are finally going outdoors again, like in the old days. North America is full of food treasures that are waiting for us to find and bring joy to our taste buds. From wild mushrooms to berries and herbs, you can find so many possible ingredients that will definitely limit the need to purchase from stores. In fact, some of these foods are packed with even more nutrition than their commercial counterparts since they are completely free of chemicals and pesticides that can do more harm than good. No, forager would tell you that they completely live off the land but will definitely say that they have saved quite a handsome amount of money by doing so.

As long as you're a human being, you have what it takes to become a forager. With a little bit of training and knowledge, you can become incredibly self-sufficient and learn skills that you can apply to your daily life activities as well, such as cooking and cleaning. So, if you're ready to become a forager or simply looking for a hobby, this book will serve you well. We start off by talking about what foraging is in detail and how it started and evolved thousands of years ago. From there, we move on to modern foraging and how you can get started right away. Since we live in the 21st century, we have to follow the rules and regulations of our time as we cannot simply forage wherever and whenever we see fit. Even though most people are familiar with foraging, it is not something that fits into the norms of modern society, especially in urban cities. Picking up apples or berries from a park may seem harmless, but you may end up breaking the law and spend some time behind the bar for different charges depending on where you are, so you have to learn the new rules fast.

Once you're familiar with the rules in your town or city, you can begin looking up what fruits, nuts, and seeds are easily found there. Some people usually forage for specific items like herbs, which they can easily grow at home as well. While others love trying out new ingredients and create exciting dishes exclusively using foraged ingredients. So much so that you can now find restaurants around the world offering unique menus that will definitely test your curiosity. With social media and YouTube, we have access to so much going on in the world. Since foraging isn't exactly normal in the modern world, it is definitely making some noise in the social atmosphere with bloggers, celebrities, scientists, and even survival instructors like Bear Grylls introducing foraging to the world directly or indirectly. We all know how news can spread and what do you know, we have a movement on the rise. There is so much more coming, but in this book, we'll be focusing on foraging as it is now and how you can become one.

Chapter 1

Foraging

Foraging is the act of searching, gathering, and harvesting food that grows in the wild for sustenance. For our distant ancestors who evolved as foragers and hunters, it was a way of life and necessary activity for survival. However, as we slowly evolved and gave rise to agriculture and commercial food production, one of our most basic skills slowly disappeared and now remains as nothing more than a recreational activity for a small group of people. In developed nations like the United States, foraging is almost non-existent unless you call looking for a midnight snack in the fridge hunting and gathering.

Even though the practice of foraging has been around for 95 percent of human existence, the last few decades of industrial farming have dominated the food market. Foraging is now limited only to people who live a self-sufficient life due to social, environmental and economic consciousness. So, unless you grew up on a farm or close to a forest, you've probably never seen or heard of anyone foraging apart from maybe a few homeless people dumpster diving. While mass production of food solves a huge problem, especially with the advancement in technology and mega supply chains to make it readily available anywhere you go, we might just lose another human trait or basic skill. If you think about it, the majority of Americans don't know basic skills like cooking, cleaning, building, or using tools, something that would probably make our ancestors weep.

People generally see convenience as a good thing, solving problems and saving time. It's not that all convenience is bad, but relying too much on many modern conveniences is suppressing our human ways. This causes more harm than good affecting a person's ability to do things themselves. Even convenience has a price you pay, be it money, time, or health in the case of convenience food. However, what was once a way of life isn't completely lost but is now more of a hobby. Some people like sports. Others like to travel, cook, paint, ready, and do normal recreational activities. Then comes people who do things a bit differently, like living off the grid, growing their own food, and living a self-sufficient life.

While this may seem strange living in the world as it is today, it is just what humans have done for thousands of years. Foraging may be considered odd in the modern world, but if you think about it, relying on food provided by nature. However, the gathering of plants, fruits, animals, and birds, rather than spending money to buy all of it does sound like an intriguing idea. This doesn't mean you stop going to the supermarket but rather reduce the amount of money you spend, thereby getting some things from nature for free. Why buy an orange when you could walk or drive by an orchard or an orange grove as they call it and pick a few, but not too man, though. You don't want to collect more than you need because then it's not really foraging.

Furthermore, megacities and structures are causing a lot of trouble around the country with wildfires, climate change, poor air quality, and invasive species. Apart from this, too much convenience in food options is causing public-health challenges such as obesity, diabetes, and heart diseases at the community level. This is because an effort to obtain food has been taken out of the picture, and unlike before, humans don't really have to do much to have a meal. While there is no single solution to this problem, the ancient practice of foraging can make a difference with people focusing on having just enough rather than hoarding and stocking your fridge. It's time we go back to the days when food was about simply living daily. The ways of our ancestors may be old and considered unorthodox in our time, but seeing generations have come and gone since then, it was definitely an effective practice of sourcing food.

What has changed since then is that we are not as connected with the natural environment as we used to be. Today, we are more focused on getting good grocery deals at the convenience store and Black Friday sales during which we will spend the night outside just to get our hands on consumer goods. When it comes to food, people hardly talk about real food like meat, vegetables, and fruits. Instead, they talk about fast food like pizza, sushi, and doughnuts, along with anything other easily accessible foods. However, times are changing with different groups of people dedicating their lives to bringing back our old ways in life. The tiny house movement has already found its way back to society, with thousands of people downsizing to manage their expenses better. Why not take it one step further and eliminating some, if not all, food expenses by foraging? It feels like connecting with our past is the only way to shape a brighter future, which is why humans are taking a step back.

Our food system has come a long way in the last century alone, thanks to industrialization. Today, food grows on big farms, and we never really see how it comes to be. This is one of the reasons why we never develop the interest to learn as well. Ask an average American in an urban area if they've ever seen food growing out of the ground, and they'll most probably say no. Back in the day, there was more to food than basic energy requirements for survival. People had a connection with their kitchen and interacted with each other. Cooking was much adventurous back then and considered to be the last step to a meal's journey. Today, it consists of bringing out ingredients from the fridge, some cutting, and dicing and into the pan. While just over a century ago, kids would pick up fresh ingredients from nature, and men would go hunting for deer or wild goose. Even though this was time and energy-consuming, it brought humans close to nature, if anything. Not to mention, the added burnt calories to stay fit and not worry about a few extra at dinner. Modern ways might be efficient, but they are driving us away from basic knowledge. For instance, you could pick wild plants that are edible and nutritious, as well as those that could give you a bad stomach or worse. That's the problem right there. Humans used to have detailed knowledge about food and plants, so much so that they passed it down to their children and younger generations. However, it doesn't have to be this way, at least not all completely. But before we get into more details, let us briefly look at the history of foraging and how our ways have changed since then.

The Evolution of Foraging

Like many animals, humans also forage and have been doing so for thousands of years. However, back then, there wasn't much choice in the matter. The earliest human beings on Earth got their food in two ways; foraging for plants and fruits, and hunting down animals. This food included berries from bushes, wild greens, mushrooms, and meat from small or large animals. Over the years, they got really good at it and could recognize which fruits and plants were edible and which were poisonous. Moreover, with continuous practice, they were able to tell what could be found in different seasons and how to manage their resources better until then. Different people from around the world developed their own ideas or ways, but what we do know is that humans communicated verbally, accumulated knowledge, and pass it on to younger generations.

Before farming was invented, foragers had different subsistence requirements. Temporary shelters were common, and people were always on the move in small groups with limited contact with others. Food diets depended on the environment and conditions people were in but was well-balanced depending on the season. With agriculture slowly becoming the new normal, humans began to settle down in one place where they could populate and live out their lives with trading networks and complex societies. However, this did not necessarily equate to improved health since, in the beginning, farming was limited to a single or at best two crops. So, the population which had grown did not have the balanced diet the previous generations had before them. The same way, farming also led to the raising of livestock. While they contributed to being a food source for larger groups of people, they also caused a lot of diseases and parasites as a result of waste.

Many historians believe that foraging was one of the leading activities that made us what we are today. With the change in seasons, survival became difficult due to which humans had to move to find other food sources. The nomadic lifestyle led to the development of other traits such as loss of hair, smaller intestines, larger brains, and walking on two feet. The most important development, however, was the ability to communicate with each other. So, we can say that it was our search for food to survive that essentially kick-started our evolution. Eventually, this led to the man's ability to control fire to cook meat and plants more than a million years ago. This ability is one of the key distinguishing features that separate us from animals.

Because of the nutrition provided by cooked food, our intestines began to shorten, and now we don't even have to chew that much anymore. Eating together gave rise to the concept of society and inter-dependence, which eventually led to settlements in the future. Over time, humans began to improve their hunting skills and developed different weapons and tools as well. By working together, they began to devise creative ways to not only hunting but gathering food spread over large areas. So, instead of individuals collecting multiple food items, groups of people began collecting single food items and exchanging them. So, you don't need to be a historian to know that foraging has been around since prehistory. Many of us have watched movies and cartoons based on the lives of Stone Age people and Caveman, so we can't really deny the idea of looking for food to eat.

As humans moved from caves and villages to suburbs and urban cities, foraging slowly became a lost and forgotten skill among the masses. Even with efforts by celebrities and important figures in the late 70s worked temporarily before people realized they could simply drive by the store to buy mushrooms and herbs with little effort. You can imagine this is the 70s we're talking about where we were still finding our way around technology. In 2020, why even bother going to the store when you can bring the store home to you? Even though this is how it still is almost everywhere, we are seeing some sparks here and there that may just bring back foraging into our lives. We've heard the saying, "modern problems require modern solutions," but are modern solutions really working? With living expenses climbing through the roof, people from all walks of life are slowly finding ways to save money. Thousands of people are downsizing and cutting down expenses any way they can, which includes cooking at home and growing their own food as well.

A Rising Trend

Foraging is an eco-activity that can be done anywhere from parks, forests, gardens, and even in your backyard. Many people don't know where to start, which is why they never take it seriously, but our world is changing so much that it almost feels as if we're going back in time. People are rapidly moving out of big cities and into rural areas. Urbanization isn't as appealing as it has been in the five decades, so people are going back to the old ways. In the same way, adventurers like Bear Grylls and Ray Mears are making foraging incredibly popular on television by not only teaching survival skills but also introducing different plants for food and other purposes. When was the last time you used marsh samphire, hogweed, sea beet, and ramsons in your meal? The answer is not only never, but with an addition of, "Never heard of these ingredients before." Many renowned chefs claim that food from the wild tastes much better than our everyday processed food.

In fact, a two Michelin star restaurant named Noma in Copenhagen, Denmark, is leading the way to commercial foraging. The Scandinavian restaurant serves delicacies served from ingredients that are only found in the wild in different seasons. Many bakeries and bars have also picked up the trend serving pine cones, wild-mushroom pies, and deserts. Chefs in the US are also using foraged ingredients to add fresh and exciting flavors to menus. With sustainable models and practices imprinted on their menus, they use indigenous produce with a sense of adventure and creativity. The idea is to bring diners close to nature by introducing a blend of different flavors and ingredients. Let us take a look at some chefs and restaurants from around the country that are using foraged ingredients to serve customers.

Dan Barber, Blue Hill Stone Barns, New York, U.S.

Dan Barber is an acclaimed chef and entrepreneur who runs his restaurant in New York called Blue Hill Stone Barns. The restaurant is popular for its use of exotic produce along with 80 acres of farmland for livestock, plants, nuts, and herbs. The chefs at the restaurant forage for ingredients they use to cook for their customers.

What's more incredible is that they do not use force-feed grain to feed and fatten livestock, especially geese, but allow them to eat off the land by foraging for acorns, figs, and lupin bush seeds.

Karlos Baca, Taste of Native Cuisine, Colorado, United States

Karlos Baca is an American chef and activist who does not consider foraging a trend or a hobby, but a way of life for Native Americans. His food comes from the land he is on, which means that he uses local ingredients found in where he is cooking at that time. He also excludes commonly found ingredients such as flour, sugar, and dairy. Instead, he uses ingredients much closer to his heritage, including sweet potato, wild mushrooms, chokecherries, and elk, among others.

Patrick Hamilton, Sonoma County Mushroom Association Wild Mushroom Camp, California, U.S.

Patrick Hamilton, better known as Mycochef, is a mushroom foraging enthusiasts. The veteran has been cooking mushrooms for over 40 years and loves to share his ideas, recipes, and experiences. One of the unique learning experiences is to identify different types of mushrooms like porcini, dyers' mushrooms, and golden chanterelles, among others. Hamilton is one of the key educators at ForageSF in San Francisco. His sense of humor and can-do attitude attracts people from all over the world as he demonstrates how to identify mushrooms safely.

Eddy Leroux, Restaurant Daniel, New York, U.S.

Eddy Leroux is a chef at Restaurant Daniel in New York. He, along with Tama Matsuoka, another forager, work together to find and serve meals with unknown and exotic ingredients. These include leaves, stems, and petals along with anise hyssop and sprigs. Moreover, he introduced welcome bags filled with nettles and rose thorns. What's interesting is that the menu at the restaurant featured items that changed all year round. In fact, some of his most challenging items are only available for a few days out of the years due to which food enthusiasts make reservations much earlier than normal. You can also find some of his best recipes in their book, Foraged Flavor.

Alex Almazan

Alex Almazan is a Serbian YouTuber who resides in the US. His channel revolves around cooking in the wild with the use of organic, foraged, and home-grown ingredients. Apart from ingredients, he also uses minimal tools and open fires in his cooking as well as traditional brick-lined ovens for baking. Today, the channel has millions of subscribers and features some of the most popular American recipes made from naturally sourced ingredients.

An Emerging Need

These are just a few of many people who are playing their role in bringing back the practice. In the modern era, nothing gets past us thanks to digital access to information. It only takes a picture or video to go viral, which may bring about a mega change in our lives. Who knows, foraging might become a common activity like it used to be. It won't come as a surprise to anyone that our current global food systems are leaning towards industrialization and duplication of diets in different countries. For example, you can find Pakistani mangoes in New York grocery stores during Christmas, so why would consumers bother to care about where food is grown or wait for the right season to enjoy? For starters, one good reason would be having to pay an unreasonable amount of money for fruit just because it's out of season. There's a lesson we can learn from developing countries in Asia and Africa, from where many of our everyday food items are imported. Locals wait for seasonal food items, unlike in developed countries where consumer demands are driving all-year-round production due to which over 40 percent of produce goes to waste according to a study by NasDaily.

A handful of organizations dominate the food world. As a result, we have no control over vital resources like food and housing, especially with the increasing number of waste and still millions with needs unmet. With regulations set to favor these industries, consumers have to pay the price set for different food products even they may exceed the price of the production by a huge margin. You would think that these unsold items might be donated to the poor or needy, but they are rather discarded as waste that only creates more problems. Probably the only good thing that came out of it were freegans; people who reject consumerism and seek help from their environment to survive and reduce waste in the process by living off discarded goods. We all have a bit of freeganism in our veins, and marketers have been using this for years to trigger sales and generate revenue. This may not be conventional foraging, but you can find thousands of people who dumpster dive near restaurants, grocery stores, and food factories for edible food. So, there isn't just one way of finding a no-cost meal, and if you follow the dictionary definition of foraging, dumpster diving definitely counts. While this may sound like something poor or homeless people would do, you would be amazed to learn that this is actually a movement to counter climate change and waste. As a result, many cities, including New York and Los Angeles, are bringing back the old practice to solve a lot of problems, be it human health, nature, or economic crisis. As we read on, we will discover what has changed so far and how you could become a forager as well.

Foraging as a Profession

Most people think that foragers are hippies or extremists that simply live off the land. So, you can imagine the looks on their face when they learn that people are actually making money from foraging. As surprising at this sound, some professional foragers work for restaurants, own a sustainable business, or even provide outdoor education, including scout craft and bushcraft. When it comes to the food industry, wild ingredients fetch top dollar at fine-dining restaurants. Recent trends suggest that farm-to-table dining is slowly transitioning into field-to-table dining since food enthusiasts are looking to experience meals made from items such as wild mushrooms and forest green salads. Professionals foragers spend their days in different, possibly even extreme conditions, searching and gathering food in the wild to earn thousands of dollars. Who would have thought that foraged ingredients could fall under fine-dining in the same league as caviar, truffle, rhubarb, and scallops? Some professional foragers offer training courses that cover a range of topics such as identification of plants, seasonal harvesting, foraging laws, and ethical considerations, herbal medicine, and DIY ideas as well.

Chapter 2

Why Forage?

A lot of people question the need for foraging in the modern world. These people are those who have become a victim of commercialization and consumerism. The truth is they're not really to blame as we move into an era with technology aiming to automate, facilitate, duplicate, or speed up existing products or services. Think about it; we still do things the same way we do. For example, in the 70s, we made calls using our wired telephones. Today, we still make calls but with the use of smartphones.

In the same way, we still pay for everything we need. Back then, we only had the option to pay by cash, but now, almost all transactions are cashless. Now, when you talk about food, we still eat meat, vegetables, and fruits. The only difference is that over a century ago, you wouldn't have visited a supermarket to buy all this. The question is, why forage when everything is easily available around us? The answer to this question is far more complex than one would imagine. People do things for different reasons; they have different needs, lives, and hobbies that drive their actions. It's easy to say that people forage so they can enjoy a free meal, but no one asks why they needed to look for a free meal in the first place.

Moreover, not everyone is about that 9-5 life our economies are desperately pushing us to become. Some of us find the time to interact with our environment to experience new tastes, colors, patterns, smells, and a stress-free feeling. We understand that modern people look for more convincing reasons, so we'll get into that as well. Plants, nuts, and seeds found naturally are high in nutrients, vitamins, minerals, and, most importantly, without pesticides. This is one of the most important differences between shopping from your local store and foraging; no added chemicals. What's more amazing is that when you get to learn about foraging, you are bound to explore so many new and exciting types of plants, nuts, and seeds that you could never find or know to look for at the store. Sometimes, we walk past edible food without even knowing it. This is because many food items are not commercially available due to supply and demand making decisions. So, what's the point of having pine nuts, Morel, and chicken of the woods in a store if no one knows about them? As a result, consumers miss out on unique flavors and stick to the same routine food they eat all year round. Many of these plants, such as mullein leaves, serve great medicinal purposes, but no one will talk about it; otherwise, the pharmaceutical industry would definitely take a hit.

Benefits of Foraging

The benefits of foraging are more than you might think. However, you will need a lot of information and to learn as much as possible about what you might find out there. So, let's dig right into why you should add foraging as a leisure or recreational activity in your life.

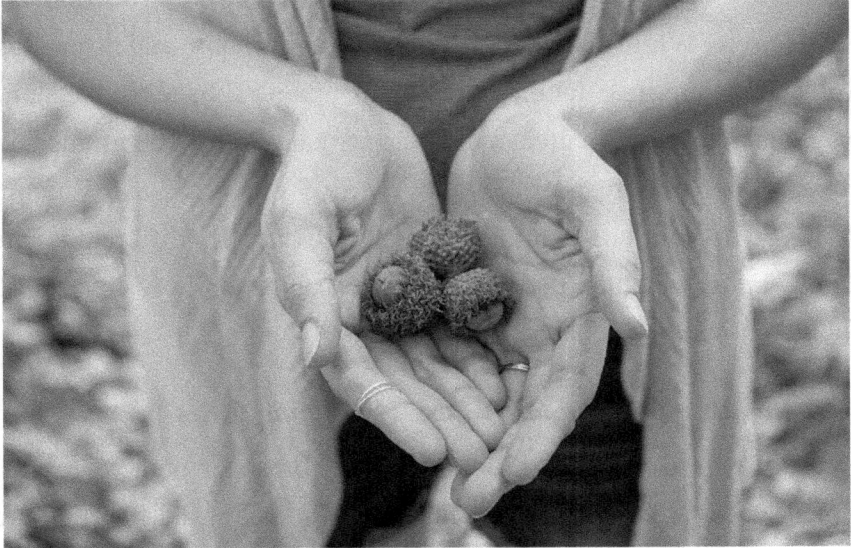

Foraging Takes You Outside

Most of us have a busy work schedule due to which we hardly find any time for ourselves. We spend our time in huge buildings on a desk all day only to come home and sleep for more of the same next day. Foraging may be just what you need to get out for some fresh air away from the noise, traffic, and people as well. If you live in New York, for example, you can easily find a local part to spend some time during lunch. All it takes is 20-30 minutes from your busy schedule to grab a bag and pull up some information from the internet regarding edible plants that are common in your area. Fireweed and Dandelions are found throughout the Northern Hemisphere.

More Nutrients Than Your Average Food Items

Many wild plants are more nutritious than cultivated plants. For example, Chenopodium Album, commonly known as wild spinach, Fat Hen or White Goosefoot, packs more protein and iron than Spinach, and more calcium and Vitamins than cabbage. In the same way, the dock leaf is a great substitute for kale as just 100 grams will cover 80 percent of your daily allowance of Vitamin C and Vitamin A. If you do your homework, you can easily identify different plants along, know whether they're safe to consume or how much you should eat without causing any problems.

Foraging Can Be Done Anywhere - Including Cities

You don't need to be close to farmland, forest, or park to forage. Green spaces are found in every major city, so taking a different route than usual to explore a different area might serve you well in finding edible food. You can also look up green spaces on Google Maps to check, and if they're close to where you are, you can easily walk or cycle for a more exciting adventure. If you're in Chicago, you can find a variety of edible plants on your way, including Butterfly Weed, Wild Quinine, and Pale Purple Coneflower.

Foraging Puts Your Taste Buds To Work

Once you get into foraging, you are bound to try out exciting new flavors you've never had before. Eating the same food can get boring over time. Ready-made meals and takeaways are fine once in a while due to intense workload and no spare time to cook. As a result, we end up eating the same food, which is really sad considering the options available. Just by walking on the street, you may come across new plants and fruits that you have never tasted before, exciting your taste buds and making you happy. Food is a great mood changer, and what better way to lift your mood if it's the food you did not have to pay for.

Foraging Is Educational

Learning about food is something everyone individual should be interested in. After all, it is our means of survival. However, this doesn't mean that you must go to college to do this; learning about wild plants can be done anywhere and anytime. All you'll need is a reference book like this one and a sense of adventure to take you outside. Plus, there's no exam at the end of the day apart from maybe putting your cooking and baking skills to test. If you're really up to it, start simply with the basic identification of plants that are common near your location and slowly build on that.

Foraged Food Can Save You Money

Not having to pay for all your food is a great way to save money. Many foragers have saved a huge chunk of their monthly expenses by picking wild vegetables instead of buying cultivated ones at the supermarket. While this option is not very consistent since you won't find vegetables and fruits every other week, but no one would say no to cutting expenses when they can.

Foraged Food Is Eco-Friendly

When people stop buying processed food and mass-produced vegetables, they shift the demand and supply curve towards less production. Less production leads to a mass reduction in the carbon footprint. This may set back mass producers to some extent and rightly so, considering how consumerism has affected common people ever since the industrial age began. Almost 40 percent of food produced goes to waste in the US every day, which is neither donated to the needy nor sold at lower prices if it exceeds its shelf life. For example, bagged salad leaves are quite expensive, and they spoil very quickly. As a result, they end up going to waste and damage the environment inevitably. Using foraged leaves can not only save you a lot of money in a year but also reduces waste and overproduction to help save the environment. Many fruits bought from stores often spoil quickly and, as a result, are thrown out as waste. Foraging requires time and effort to pick out fruits, so people are less likely to take more than they need and even less likely to let them spoil and go to waste.

Foraged Food Makes Great Drinks

If you know your way around fermentation and have a hobby of making your own booze, foraging is a great option to add unique flavor to alcoholic wines and beer. Wildflowers, leaves, berries, and roots are abundant in nature to add excitement to your taste buds plus, they limit the need to purchase processed alcohol from stores. Great options include dandelion root beer and elderflower champagne since they require minimum technical skills to make.

Foraged Food Is Great For Medicine

Foraging is not just a way of obtaining food. For thousands of years, humans have used plants for natural remedies and herbal medicine. Garden herbs, weeds, and plants of the earth have served as a veritable treasure for us for millennia. These plants have been used for different purposes, including disinfecting wounds, fighting stomach and headaches, growing long hair, and other cosmetic purposes. For example, wild roses are packed with Vitamin C, so next time you're on your way back from your morning run, grab a few to make tea. This will help with muscle repair and general recovery from fatigue. Natural remedies and immunity boosters can replace the need for supplements that cost a lot and require a prescription as well.

Foraging Connects You With Nature

Not a lot of people notice that their curiosity level peaks when they're outside. This is most definitely our basic human instinct to explore kicking in without us even realizing it. Foraging is a great all-round activity if you think about it. It's physical, requires strategy and planning, and at the end of the day, it's literally fruitful.

Foraging Expands Your Menu

A lot of us find ourselves cooking the same meals a day in and out, which can get boring over time, hence, developing the urge to eat out more often. Many foraged items are not commonly found in supermarkets, so using them adds new flavor to your food, thus, bringing more excitement to your kitchen and pantry. Plus, it's not like others aren't doing it. You can find hundreds of recipes from all around the world with foraged ingredients like wild mushrooms, dandelions, and wild spinach.

Foraging Helps Support Self-Sufficient Living

For those looking to live a self-sufficient life, foraging is among the key activities to get you there. Not everyone can grow food at home, but with nature almost all around us, you don't really need to. Thousands of people are using the latest technology to engage in some of our most ancient practices. You can find people living off the grid, generating their own power, raising their own livestock, and moving around the country to live a different kind of lifestyle. Not having to buy food every time is a great way to be self-sufficient, although not everyone can say that. It's all a matter of perspective and what self-sufficiency means to them.

Foraging Counters Consumerism

It's been a long-standing idea that a person's wellbeing and happiness depends on obtaining consumer goods and material possessions. Now, the key here is the word obtaining, which is usually with money. While money is the way our world works today, we have gone from wanting to have just enough to wanting as much as possible. If you think about it, food was as much about the experience as the meal itself. Foraging is one of the players in the game, bringing people back to a simpler way of life.

Hazards of Foraging

Foraging has its downside live everything else, most of which can easily be avoided. However, hazards are everywhere, but when it comes to foraging, they are usually faced by newbie foragers that don't really have the experience or the full information. The following are some of the major risks of foraging;

Getting Arrested

Law is what separates us from the animals as they say, and like everything else, there are active foraging laws and regulations that not most people are unaware of. You'd think you're simply picking fruit or plant only to end up in jail for not knowing that it was a protected species. Moreover, it is illegal to forage on a person's property with permission, and many parks around the country also forbid gathering plants. However, a few exceptions have been made from time to time for people who have no other way to survive. Plus, there are no limits on how much you can forage, so there's no way to tell when you're over-foraging.

Getting Sick or Poisoned

Not every plant you find in the wild is edible. Some are extremely poisonous, while others might make you mildly sick or cause allergies. Whatever the case, many foragers mistake poisonous plants for safe ones, and often end up in the emergency room or worse. In fact, even experts with years of experience aren't immune to the dangers. Moreover, usually, plants that are found close to the living population are edible but may still make your sick if they have been having contaminated by chemicals, animal waste, or pesticides.

Lack of Knowledge

You might find great plants, vegetables, nuts, or seeds in the wild but not know what to do with them. Experienced foragers know that it's not just about finding edible food in the wild, but how to eat it. A lot of these food items can taste awful if not prepared correctly, so it's a good idea to do some research. Otherwise, it's time, effort, and produce wasted just because of not knowing how to use it.

Damaging the Environment

Not everyone knows how much harvesting is ok without killing off the plant completely. Newbie foragers often end up destroying the whole plant just to have more than normal. Many foragers have damaged delicate environments by simply walking on them, which displaces the topsoil, crushes the plant, and even promotes habitat inundation.

Foraging vs. Farming

While there is no denying that farming and agriculture have opened doors for the human race and allowed us to flourish, it has also taken a lot of us in terms of knowledge and skill. Today, we hardly know anything about nature unless our field of study specifically allows us to. So, apart from farmers, botanists, biologists, and environmentalists, not many people could recognize, let alone know how to find or grow plants. Taking away nothing from farming, which has been one of the greatest ideas mankind has ever had and the reason for the growth of civilization, foraging shouldn't have ended. With technology on the rise, humans are becoming weaker but not in a Terminator movie kind of way but our ability to do things ourselves. While hierarchy brought order to the society, which boosted efficiency, complete dependency on mass-produced goods has caused not only division in society but also controlled the market. Profit is the aim of every business, but regulations in the pricing of products have been extremely poor in all goods and services. Only in the United States is healthy living more expensive as compared to living off processed and fast food. Fresh produce is dependent on manual labor and resources, which is why the average cost of food daily is around $42, which tells you everything you need to know. So, every month, every household spends $1200-$1500 on food alone, which is a massive amount. There are lots of ways you can save though including growing food yourself, and foraging as well. So, with a bit of effort and patience, you could save hundreds of dollars on a monthly recurring basis. Apart from this, foragers and non-foragers usually have a different lifestyle, and it has much more to do than what they eat.

Foragers are usually fit and eat a different variety of food. Even though the reason for this is obvious, we'll explain why. While strolling down the park or riding a bike, you constantly burn calories and exercise your muscles. Moreover, natural food sources are rich in proteins and vitamins that boost your immunity. Plus, with expenses piling up, not everyone can afford to eat healthily. Since foragers live off the land, they don't have to worry about money to buy healthy food or get a gym membership. Many studies say that people who spend time outdoors are more mentally fit, and it does not just have to do with the extra fresh air. Humans were never meant to stay in one place, so connecting to nature is simply our basic human instinct. Secondly, many foragers are self-sufficient people who do not rely a lot on purchased food; neither do they plant and harvest their own crops. Unlike farming, foraging is a seasonal or occasional activity, so foragers don't put in as many hours as farmers. While farming offers a consistent supply of food, foraging is more about living according to the natural order of the land. Foragers live a life that does not differentiate between the rich and the poor. One of the biggest problems in mass-produced food is segregation between different classes of people. Food in the wild is equally available to everyone. In fact, foragers are more likely to enjoy luxury ingredients that the majority of people would have to pay ridiculous sums of money to eat. There is no doubt that farming creates job opportunities for millions, if not billions of people around the world. However, at the end of the day, people use most of their money on food and utilities anyway. While this isn't exactly a bad thing, it's also not as if farmers are ruling the world today.

Another concern that foraging usually brings about is the foraged food itself, and it's not even about being poisonous. Most of the time, perfectly edible wild food may end up being contaminated with bacteria, chemicals, and diseases, which is something many foragers usually ignore in their early days. Plus, nature is not only home to delicious food but also wild animals and plants. North America is no stranger to snakes and poisonous animals that live in the same mountains and forests where foragers aim to get their food from. Based on immediate danger, foragers don't often live a very long life span. However, with obesity, diabetes, and heart diseases making headlines in the US, foragers might actually have a better life span than average America living off processed food. Foragers like to live on their feet, so while others may think that they always worry about when their next meal or drink may come from, this is never the case. Foragers organize plans ahead to get buy, which is the reason they maintain physical and mental fitness. Having food at all times is the reason people over-eat and are stressed most of the time.

Health vs. Technology

Foragers have been known to be healthier than non-foragers, and it has nothing to do with processed food or sugar. Farmers back in the day had diets that were high in carbohydrates but low in fiber and protein. This led to an increase in body fat and slower childhood growth. Different studies also claimed that as agriculture advanced and humans limited foraging activities, they became shorter and weaker. While technology was on the rise with different tools and cultivating techniques, there was one thing farmers could not control; drought. The drought was the main reason for crop failure and famines. While food eventually became abundant as time passed by with consistent supply chains, diseases spread much more rapidly than during the time in which foragers and hunters existed. This was not only because humans began living together instead of being constantly on the move, but the domestication of animals which spread parasites and bacteria since sanitation was inadequate. While farmers grew in skills, humans that didn't stop foraging lived longer and were more immune to diseases. Even today, not a lot has changed. According to the CDC, 40 percent of adults in their 20s are obese, and 70 percent are above their normal weight and height index. So, in a millennium, we have come a long way in terms of food technology, and somehow, people are even less healthy than before. So, the question is, what hasn't changed? Is it the fact that technology advancements have focused more on speeding up food production and availability and not the food itself? If hunting and foraging made us stronger and more immune to diseases, why didn't we ensure that we allowed it to an extent? Someone once said that innovations would lead to more questions than answers, and it seems like it fits this case perfectly.

Escape from Modern Technology

In the last millennia or so, technology has progressed at an amazing rate. Thousands of inventions and advancements in communication, travel, business, and agriculture are constantly changing every small facet of our lives. While we are making new grounds everywhere and changing our lives, we are also changing ourselves and not necessarily in a good way. There was a time humans did most things themselves. Every average person was a polymath in different domains and didn't rely a lot on others to do things for them. Individuals used to build their own houses, not look for the closest construction company. The same way, getting a hot meal required a lot more work than simply ordering take out or microwaving ready-made Mac N Cheese. As a result, humans are not as skilled as they were back in the day and the following are some of the areas they have been affected in;

Attention

There is no denying that the internet and mobile technology have improved every single thing we do, whether it's in terms of time, resources, or energy. However, it is shortening our attention span. So much so, that in less than four seconds, you can go from wanting to go for a stroll in the park to playing games or binge-watching. Since we're so used to getting everything quickly, we've lost most of our patience. Foraging is one of the many activities that can improve attention spans if you take it seriously. If anything, foraging in 2020 and beyond doesn't have to be old school. Sure, you'll have to use for a smartphone for research while on the move, but this time, it'll be worth it.

Decision-Making

You need to cook dinner. What's the first thing you do? According to studies, millions of people go online to do research. While doing so, they come across thousands of options and often go for either the cheapest or the most convenient option to fill their craving. The internet has become a great source of advice, but when humans tend to rely heavily on anything, they no longer rely on their basic instincts to make informed decisions. Plus, the time they spent on looking up food could have been spent on literally looking at food.

Memory

Technology has given us access to a huge amount of information, which is not only accessible in real-time but can also be stored on our devices. So, how many of us really remember their daily tasks without having to look them up on sticky notes or calendars? Our reliance on technology has decreased our ability to retain information the same way the rise of self-driving cars in the near future may not require driving skills.

The fact of the matter is that technology should be promoted but not at the expense of our own abilities. Sure, it's meant to improve efficiency and facilitate humans, but this doesn't mean that we become entirely dependent on it. Just because you can call triple 24/7 roadside assistance doesn't mean you shouldn't be able to change a flat tire. The same way, just because you have food easily available at a cost everywhere doesn't mean you cannot or shouldn't sometimes forage if not always. Thousands of people across the country are doing it every day to not only save a few bucks here and there but also to remain mentally and physically fit by reconnecting with nature. Modern life involves fitting yourself into different boxes, from those with walls or wheels, be it our home, office, restaurant, or car. Staying all day indoors working or even chilling fuels anxiety and insomnia, among other things. Moreover, it's safe to say that our televisions are getting slimmer every at the same rate we're gaining inches.

Chapter 3

Foraging In The United States

Foraging is a growing activity in the United States. However, a lot of questions are raised on how to govern it on a large scale. As a result, the laws are complicated all around. Since there are federal, state, and local laws and regulations in the United States, often these regulations contradict each other. You might think that you're simply picking a fruit from a tree while strolling down the park, but in the eye of the law, you've just become a lawbreaker. Rules vary everywhere you go from jurisdiction to jurisdiction. Plus, foraging for food in the modern era isn't really considered what you might call "Normal" so picking food might make you viewed as a subversive person. If not subversive, people would definitely perceive you as a poor person or someone doing it for survival. A leisure activity won't even be the last thing they consider this. Many governing bodies and scholars consider foragers as society rebels looking to disrupt the stability of the system.

Urban Foraging Laws

Urban cities have strict and just laws governing foraging activities, especially in megacities like New York. Park department ordinance prohibits the destruction and cutting of trees as well as removing plant vegetation. So, basically, anyone would naturally assume that foraging is illegal in New York; however, that isn't exactly the case. There are no restrictions that prohibit picking fruits from trees according to the ordinance, which is more vague than broad with not enough detail or loopholes that may favor either side. So, basically, we have Schrodinger's cat situation, which means foraging is both legal and illegal, depending on the situation. However, in most cases, foragers are never given the benefit of the doubt due to the ordinance and official interpretations of it. In fact, you could have to pay up to $250 in fines if you get caught. In 1986, a New Yorker named Steve Brill, better known as "Wildman," was arrested for organizing paid foraging tours in Central Park. Officially, his crime was recorded as plucking and eating dandelion greens, which the park's commissioner didn't take well. Ultimately, his case went public and was discharged after he agreed to officially work with the parks department as a foraging tour organizer.

Not too far away in Maryland, another man Greg Visscher was fined $50 by the police for picking raspberries in a local park. His case was also dismissed since the nature of picking the raspberries wasn't clear, according to the reports. The issue with the ordinance is that it is still very raw and needs to be refined in order to really manage things better. There are tons of other examples that have made the news like an elderly man from Chicago who was fined $75 picking dandelion greens for a salad. So, you can see that many of these laws are uncaring, absurd, and uncalled for. Some of the major urban cities in America, such as Seattle, Philadelphia, New York, and Cleveland all have foraging restrictions that are more leaning towards prohibition. However, Seattle is an exception, as it is one of the few taking foraging very seriously. They started off by turning overgrown lots into large parks for locals. One of the incredible places to visit is Beacon Food Forest, which includes a variety of fruits such as pears, plums, apples, raspberries, grapes, and blueberries, along with many other options. The motive is to give back to the constituents of the major city in a unique way, and the trend is already rising in other major cities around the country. In other cities such as Baltimore, parks don't necessarily prohibit foraging but do not permit damaging grass, flora, trees, and shrubbery. However, getting permission for a limited amount is acceptable and recommended as well.

Many foragers are slowly waking up and speaking up against these insane laws. Any good forager knows better than to destroy nature, so these bans and fines are unnecessary. Sure, overharvesting can be a problem, but to prevent that, we need regulations, not complete banning of the activity. If Seattle can embrace foraging, why not other major cities like Chicago, New York, Texas, and New Jersey? New York City did eventually pick on the movement with an idea of an urban food forest away from the city on the Bronx River. This way, it would never be short of water supply and not too packed with human presence to ensure sustenance. Not to mention, it will present a great opportunity to forage vegetables, fruits, and herbs without the fear of being charged with a fine. Today thousands of residents have access to free food and medicine as a result since the ban on foraging was on land, not water. This loophole led to New York becoming one of the first major cities in the country to establish a manmade urban forest.

State Foraging Laws

State laws on foraging are far more varying, and surprisingly, it is where wild foods are abundant and rich that various agencies and bodies have placed strict restrictions to make it nearly impossible. So much, so that heavy penalties are being implemented on foragers in California. However, Alaska, the last frontier as expected, is much more open to natural and traditional use of wild resources in the rural areas. Residents are protected in other geographically diverse American states, including Arkansas, Colorado, Florida, Hawaii, Maine, and Florida. However, most of these laws aren't uniform, so foragers have to learn them if they ever decide to take their adventures out of state. Alaska is known for its recreational harvesting of wild plants, berries, and mushrooms, among other natural resources, but only for personal and non-commercial use. The only law that remains consistent anywhere you go is the prohibition of the destruction, disturbance, or removal of plants from state parks. At the same time, Colorado prohibits all foraging activities in state parks, while Florida only allows foraging not, harvesting in their parks apart from aquatic plants. Hawaii allows all foraging activities but to a certain limit to prevent over-harvesting. In Maine, foraging has been practiced for decades and is part of a long tradition in which they are calling permissive trespass of property. So, basically, if the owner of the property has no issue with people foraging off their land, then no harm is done.

Federal Foraging Laws

Conservation of land is the way to go when it comes to federal foraging laws. With that said, you can scratch off all national parks and federal lands if you are planning to forage there unless you have no problem being arrested for trespassing. However, there is another policy that actually encourages the use and enjoyment of national parks by the public with regulations, of course, set in place. This policy has been added to the Organic Act, which serves to conserve scenery, nature, historical landmarks and objects, and of course, wildlife. It is the same law which doesn't allow you to go fishing in city lakes or rivers. Our national parks and forests are managed by NPS and the U.S. Forest Service, which is a part of the Department of Agriculture. With the NPS, you don't need a permit to forage in the mountains. However, according to the Forest Service, you have to not only obtain a permit but also pay a fee to harvest forest products. So, in the end, the idea of free food by foraging goes straight out the window, but you might still have a good time.

In 2020, foraging for food is an emerging activity to boost community, nutritional education, and even some unconventional political movements. However, the sole focus of foraging is to connect with nature to understand the process and where it all comes from. Many people are considering foraging as a way of reconnecting with botanical origins of food and thereby developing different social movements including the following;

Freeganism

By definition, freeganism is an ideology of reluctance to participate in conventional ways of living and consuming resources. The movement started in the 60s in San Francisco, by a group who organized free housing, clinics and gave away rescued food to the needy. The movement is more about solidarity against consumerism and militarism rather than an act of charity. The word freegan is a portmanteau for free and vegan, and this basically explains what kind of people these are. While vegans avoid meat and animal products, freegans take it one step further by not purchasing anything to eat along with not eating meat. These people like to tread as lightly as possible by living completely, giving up all purchases. Instead, they get what they need with sharing, scavenging, and borrowing. While descendants of the Diggers have a vision of a money free society with free goods and labor, modern freegans focus on a lifestyle in which they live off free food, challenging the evils of modern society that relies on greed, waste, meaningless work and inequality. Since they never buy anything, including their food, they spend a lot less than others. Their aim is not really to save money, but by doing so, they benefit from the result of their choice to do so. Different freegans have different reasons for choosing this kind of life and here are some interesting reasons.

Human Rights

Many freegans are human right activists that are concerned about the wellbeing of farmers. They argue that just about everything sold in stores is produced in conditions that harm human beings, be it pesticide poisoning, third-world health conditions, and financial instability. The problem is that multi-national firms do not care or give back to the laborers who have made them billions of dollars but hardly live to make the average income of a common American. They believe that avoiding spending money on these systems could lead to a systematic change in which shareholders will stop hoarding most of the profits and improve the lives of the people that contribute to their revenue streams.

Environmental Concerns

Freegans are concerned about the environment. They believe that mass-produced goods and over-industrialization are the reason global warming is on the cars thanks to industrial pollution, landfilling, waste of materials and heavy use of the oil-based process, from manufacturing to shipping to distribution. So, the idea is simple; the less you shop and consume commercial products and services, the less the carbon footprint you leave. Plus, they believe if people start doing this on a large scale, they might bring about the needed change this world desperately needs.

Animal Welfare

Like Vegans and vegetarians, freegans oppose factory farms in which animal cruelty is commonly practiced. The giant farms raise millions of animals in small spaces and horrible conditions. Apart from giant farms and commercial production of livestock, freegans are also against the use of pesticides used in farming, which results in not only habitat destruction but also inundation. If anything, they believe in the old ways in which small-scale farms were common.

A Minimalist Lifestyle

Freegans believe that we weren't brought into this world simply to work and die. This is why they prefer to live a simple and minimalist life in which they choose to buy as little as they can so they can afford to work less. Many freegans do not spend on new items and live off scavenged goods. This way, they can find more time to be socially active rather than work ridiculously long hours to pay off expenses that they don't really need. Freegans like to believe that they have more in common with our hunter-gatherer ancestors than other people.

When it comes to obtaining food, freegans try to make the best use of discarded food from commercial establishments such as restaurants, hotels, and retail stores. While people may consider this as dumpster diving, there is a much more respectable term for this practice, and it is called Urban Foraging. Freegan diets revolve around food waste that is still edible and has lived past its shelf life, season or expiry as a result of overstocking or declining demand. So, freegans are foragers that don't necessary harvest food from trees and plants but rather minimalize waste by simply letting it not happen. Plus, urban foraging is not only limited to food. The same practice is applied to books, furniture, appliances, bicycles, and clothing as well. Freegans or urban foragers don't really share much in terms of sites and strategies due to the rising competition and the whole survival of the fittest regime. However, when it comes to food wastage, a lot of awareness is slowly being spread through organized public events and activities. In fact, some of the most popular media outlets, environmentalists, and celebrities such as Oprah, The New

York Times, and CNN have, on multiple occasions, spoke on the growing problem. On top of that, influencer channels such as NasDaily, Trash for the Tossers, and the Zero Waste Chef have all spoken up on the insane amount of food which goes to waste on a daily basis.

Apart from urban foraging, many freegans also participate in wild foraging. Wild foragers find and harvest food along with medicinal plants growing in their surroundings. Many of them also believe in creating their own community gardens where they can grow their own feed. Instead of using fertilizers, they use inedible food waste with composting techniques that allow them to set the right infrastructure for food production. This is what you may call an all-out act of self-sufficiency. Normally, eco-conscious people try to go off the grid to make a change to their lifestyle, but producing their own food independently is just taking it to new levels. Freegans like to share things. In fact, the ideology is based on a gift economy in which giving food and shelter to those in need in the way of doing things. Even when things are not free, a general barter system is introduced in what they call a free store. In this store, people exchange items, including food, in exchange for other items without the use of any money. When it comes to moving around, freegans walk or ride bikes as much as possible to eliminate the use of cars and buses. With a sense of community in mind, freegans like to stick together to learn and teach survival skills in their unorthodox way of living. It's not like freegans never spend money at all but that they don't spend unless they really have to when there isn't an alternative. For instance, freegans will not purchase cars to move around but won't mind using ridesharing apps like Uber. It wasn't until the housing crisis in 2007-08 that the media really paid attention to freeganism. With millions out of jobs and on the road, freeganism, which was considered to be a hobo way of living, suddenly became perceived as an attractive alternative lifestyle. More importantly, a lot of importance has been given to food waste as well, especially when it could be used to help millions of people. Food companies in the country would rather throw away 40 percent of all food produced daily rather than give it to the needy, which is one of the reasons why this social group started in the first place.

The Paleo Diet

Freeganism isn't the only social movement that is hitting the foraging world by storm. Alternative diets are making the same amount of noise in different neighborhoods, if not louder. Over the years, we have witnessed the increase in health awareness from allergies to calories. This awareness has changed the way we look at food since people are a lot more conscious of what they eat, especially with the abundance of options now available. No one really wants to have a glass of milk anymore. They want low-fat non-dairy soy milk instead. The same way people are beginning to question the bread they buy at the local bakery if it is whole-wheat and sugar-free. Not to mention the vegetarian, vegan, and Keto diet fanatics that are hitting digital media like a storm. In just the last decade, we have seen the rise in alternative diets and people choosing to live a healthier lifestyle with the removal of dairy, gluten, and meat from their menus. Becoming a vegetarian was considered a bold lifestyle choice, but veganism, which eliminates all animal by-products such as cheese, milk, butter, and eggs, takes alternative choices to new heights.

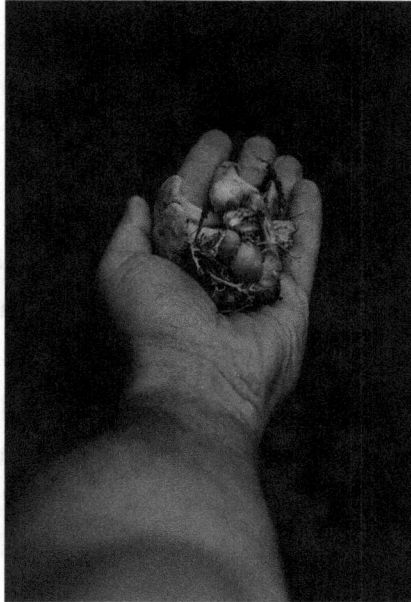

However, alternative diets have always been an important and prominent part of our history. In fact, the first-ever cultivated plants and vegetables were an alternative choice of food since our world was accustomed to foraging. With a new food source at their disposal, humans created a mixed diet, better known as the Paleolithic diet, which dates from 2.5 million to 10,000 years ago. This diet usually includes fish, lean meats, vegetables, fruits, seeds, and nuts that were obtained mostly from hunting and gathering. Dairy food came down the line, so they are not considered to be a part of this diet plan. After veganism and Keto, the Paleo diet is returning, with many people choosing to eat like early humans. The idea behind the diet is that modern diets do not match humans genetically due to which we have so many diseases. Farming largely changed what people consumed and established grains, dairy, and legumes as additional food items to the human diet, which is something that was not available way back in the day. According to Paleo diet enthusiasts, these additions were brought in much quicker than our capability to adapt to change. As a result, we now have to deal with diabetes, obesity, and heart diseases.

People who follow the Paleo diet do so for two major reasons; to lose weight and to avoid dairy. So, while you would be adding fruits, meat from different animals, vegetables, seeds, and oils, you would be avoiding wheat, oats, barley, beans, lentils, peanuts, dairy products, sugar, salt, and processed foods. While eliminating sugar, salt, and process foods are an excellent way to lose weight, the rest are among the healthiest food choices available. Just because cavemen never had them doesn't really make them bad, according to critics of the diet. However, critics of this diet have been answered with some amazing results. A number of randomized clinical trials compared different diet plans to the Paleo diet, and the results were astonishing. The trial suggests that the Paleo diet provides more benefits when compared with vegan, vegetarian, dairy, and keto. The Paleo diet led to more weight loss, improved glucose tolerance, better blood pressure control, lower cholesterol and triglycerides, and amazingly, better appetite management. People getting rid of everyday ingredients, especially salt, wheat, and sugar, shared their difficulty at first, but sooner than later, they began to enjoy the natural flavor of food. The Paleo diet has set forth a lifestyle and social movement with additions to clothing, smartphone apps, and crockery. You can also find hundreds of Paleolithic recipes, especially from Native American sources that have become best-selling books. In 2019, the Paleo market became worth $500 million, which is actually saying something. Plus, since foraging was how most of the food our ancestors ate, modern cooks try to keep many of the ingredients as original as possible.

Chapter 4

Foraging 101

If you're looking to get started as a newbie forager, the first thing you should learn is patience. It can take years to learn to identify plants, nuts, and seeds that are edible and, even more importantly, to stay away from the ones that you shouldn't eat. However, there a lot of edible plants that you can easily recognize like Apples, mushrooms, and pine cones. Nature has a lot more to offer, so there is much to learn. The trick is to start somewhere and slowly build your knowledge and expand your wild food pantry every day. Many foragers say that learning foraging is quite similar to basic farming or gardening except, you have a much bigger playground to work with. The difference is that with farming, you know what you're going to find since you'd be planting it there. Foraging is much more adventurous, and there are many more safety considerations that go with it. Before we move on to safety, let us look at some of the basic or general rules you should follow when foraging.

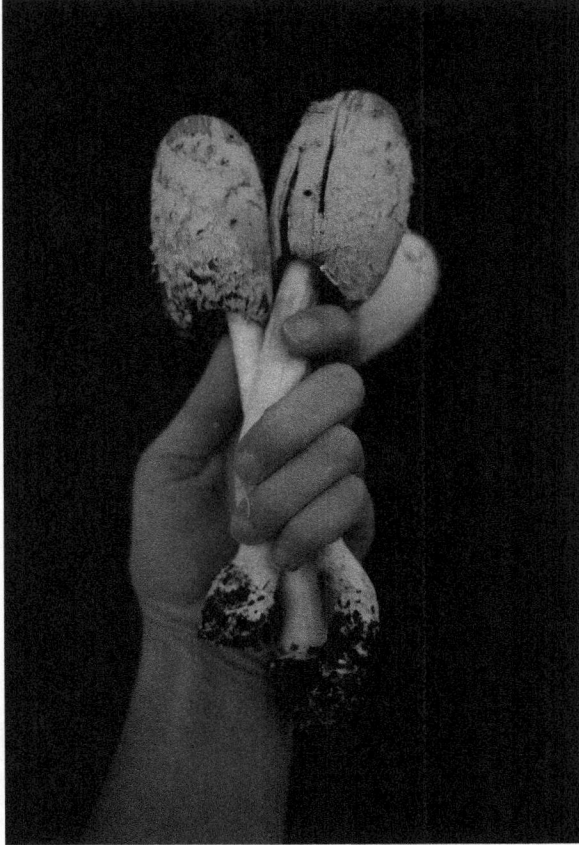

Edible But Not Really

Just because a cute little animal eats something, it doesn't mean it's safe for humans. Many plants in the wild are poisonous and can even lead to death if not taken care of at the right time.

Watch the Kids

Under no circumstances should you allow kids to eat any part of a foraged plant without your permission. While foraging is a fun activity, it could lead to a visit to a doctor if your kids are not careful.

Trust Your Nose

If you come across a plant that looks good to eat but smells weird, then there's a sign not to eat it. If you can't smell the plant as it is, try crushing a leaf and have a go-to decide.

Avoid Roadside Foraging

In many cases, foragers have to do with what they have, but if they can avoid something, they should. For instance, you should avoid or repeatedly wash roadside plants, since they have most definitely been sprayed with pesticides and been contaminated with pollutants from vehicles and animals.

Say No to Spoiled Food

Even if quick foods like berries and nuts look tempting, do not eat them if they appear to be spoiling. You could have an upset stomach or, at the very least, have to spit out the awful tasting berry immediately.

Start Small

There are tons of food items your taste buds and tummy haven't discovered yet, so start off small. You may love what you're eating, but your stomach might not feel the same way and react accordingly. It's the same as adapting to eating spicy food all of a sudden or start eating meat after a few months of the boycott. Let your stomach adapt to new food items on your menu, so as you develop your foraging skills; you also maintain a strong stomach to digest everything you eat.

If you go on the internet and look up societies across the globe that are still connected to nature, you would find that basic knowledge of plants and harvesting is essential. While this knowledge was quite common a century go even in the US, it has been lost today for well-known reasons. Since that kind of life doesn't exist in the modern world, that knowledge is deemed pretty useless overall. What we do know is that if you find yourself lost, stranded and hungry in the forest or park, you probably wouldn't know what to do. No normal person has the skill, knowledge, or experience of living off the land. Even with farming well known and practiced around the world, if you're not a farmer, chances are you have zero plant, fruits, nuts, and seed knowledge apart from which supermarket you could get all these from. If you are going to call yourself a forager in the near future, the first thing you'll need to learn about plants that are:

Common

Every forager needs to be aware of the plants that are commonly found where they are or relatively close to it. Without this, you really don't have much to start off with since it's not like you're going to walk on the road and suddenly find potatoes.

Easily Identified

If you'd see a tomato or a mango, you'd easily identify both. However, it's very unlikely you find either in a forest in North America. Instead, you're more likely to find prickly pears, berries, and wild spinach along with a lot of plants that look alike but are completely different from each other and are often poisonous as well.

Easily Processed

For beginners, it is better to start off easy. This means looking for plants that don't require a lot of work, whether it's in harvesting, cooking, or even fermenting. Try to find food that you can consume immediately or almost immediately. When it comes to fruits, you simply need to wash them, and you're good to go. With most vegetables and plants, just a few minutes in the pan with some season is enough. If you find something that requires time when you're hungry at that moment, it's not exactly a waste but not really helpful either.

Available

Newbie foragers should look to options that are available for longer periods of time. Sure, you can wait for seasonal fruits and vegetables, but it's better to gain more experience by regularly being out there. This way, you not only become good at what you do but prepare to take on new wild challenges.

When you connect deeply with nature by foraging, you get to bring new life to your taste buds. However, one bad choice and you might see yourself in the emergency room or worse so, knowledge is essential. Even if you do recognize a plant, you have to ensure by checking again that your identification is correct. Even after years of experience, some foragers say that they can still be surprised by what they find in the wild and also have trouble recognizing exactly what they're looking at. When eating foraged food, it's not just about looking for food that is safe in terms of whether it's poisonous or not, but also in terms of contamination. A dog could easily mark its territory on a plant that looks absolutely delicious to consume right away, or you might find some incredibly tempting dandelions on a busy city road. So, you should know when to prepare or stop yourself. People have spent years training themselves to add new flavors to their plates from nature safely. So much so, that you'd be surprised to see what they have on their menu. For example, wild strawberries are practically invisible from human height, but you'd still find them in deserts or salads made by experienced foragers. In fact, any good forager is well aware of what to find in different seasons, and they actually look forward to bringing home these seasonal fruits and vegetables when the time comes.

Foraging is like supermarket shopping except that not everything is always available and the fact that you don't have to pay for anything you get. However, this doesn't mean that you'll always come back with a basket full of food from your foraging expedition. The same way, just because you forage doesn't mean you'll completely stop going to the supermarket every now and then. The only difference is that there might be a few times that you actually find a free alternative in the wild, so you end up saving some money for something else. Another quality of a good forager is that they will never take more than they need or trespass where they're not welcome. This means that they always leave some for the next time they visit and ensure the plant is never destroyed. If you dig up plants completely, you're going to kill them, but snipping off just a few leaves or picking fruit does no harm since the plant will continue to grow. Moreover, always be considerate that wildlife is dependent on the food that grows in forests, gardens, or parks, so always leave some for them. They can't go to the supermarket like humans can if they run out. Today, only a hand full of people in the western world knows anything about foraging apart from homeless people dumpster diving in order not to starve. While it's perfectly fine not to be an expert or anything, basic knowledge could make a difference to your life, and it's nothing that is too difficult to try. If you make an effort, you might find yourself living a complete human life as it was meant to be along with all the modern perks of society.

A Forager's Toolkit

Suppose you have developed a keen interest in foraging or just looking for a hobby to have a meal with foraged ingredients. Newbie foragers usually buy into the idea that all it takes is a stroll to the park and a "can do" attitude. While getting your hands dirty isn't always a bad thing, there's a lot more in the dirt that you might not want to get your hand on. Ask any forager, and they'd tell you what fun it is walk in the woods, a nearby park, or a garden to collect your next meal. With that said, not everything you find is edible, and even if it is, it doesn't mean you should just grab and pull. There is the right way to forage, and there's the savage way that disregards the rules or basic harvesting ethics, thereby disrupting not only property but also the plant itself. Any avid forager knows that they have to plan their day of foraging according to what they intend to find. It's not always going in blind for them, since they're aware of what they're going to find out there. It's just about when and where they're going to find it is the most intriguing part of the journey. With that said, foragers, put together and carry a tool kit packed with essential items that they'll need to not only bring back the loot but also help with plucking, disinfecting, and cleaning. A basic toolkit can be divided into three categories; transport containers, picking aids, first aid, and other things. Each item serves a purpose and highly depends on the hunt at that specific time. For instance, you won't go looking for mushrooms with a pair of scissors. Sure, we all love to improvise, but it never hurts to do something right. Let us get into the details;

Transport Containers

Transport containers are the single most important thing to have when foraging. Sure, foraged food is obviously the reason for all the trouble, but there needs to be a way to transport the loot. The containers you take with you will vary on what you're expecting to bring back home. Different types of transport containers include;

Plastic Shopping Bags

You can easily find plastic shopping bags at home, whether they're from your last takeout or trip to the grocery store. They are perfect for storing large quantities of plants such as grape leaves, wild mustard, and mallow and they are also great for carrying fruits or nuts like apples, almonds, and oranges. Even though plastic bags aren't eco-friendly, using them to forage is a great alternative to throwing them in the trash.

Basket

Experienced foragers often like to do things the classic way. Baskets are commonly used as a storage or an overflow container. They have handles that make them easy to carry around as compared to shopping bags. You can also find a variety of baskets, including folding kinds or one which doubles as a backpack so you can use both hands. Baskets are much more durable than bags as well, even though they may not always deteriorate after some time. Plus, the more you forage, the more you'll have to carry, and it's not really to carry heavy baskets across long distances.

Covered Containers

Often you'd come across delicate items that can get crushed easily if you keep them in a basket or a plastic bag. Covered containers like plastic boxes are perfect for keeping soft fruits like grapes, apricots, and figs as well as delicate flowers. Apart from delicate items, many flowers, and plants, like prickly pears, often have thorns or sharp ends that may tear up plastic bags easily.

Backpacks

In many cases, all you need is a good backpack. Backpacks have plenty of pockets so you can keep different food items, especially small ones like wild berries and nuts. They are extremely comfortable to transport, and you can carry them anywhere you go safely.

Sandwich Bags

If you are one of that do-it-right kind of people, sandwich bags come in handy for those tiny food items that you forage. These include seeds, pine nuts, and capers. Sandwich bags make them easier to find in a large bag when collecting multiple items. Plus, you can always make a sandwich on your trip and use the bag later on.

Freezer Bags

Freezer bags aren't used much often by foragers, but they work well with large items that don't fit in a sandwich bag. Plus, they are sealed at the top, which not only makes them relatively airtight but also stops food items from falling out.

Picking Aids

It is safe to say that as a forager, you just cannot pick everything by hand. It doesn't matter how good you are; sometimes your fingers just won't cut it. Besides, you may damage the plant if you forcefully try to harvest it. Picking aids can be used to increase picking efficiency and reduce the time to pick things as well. The man became best friends with tools long before he did with dogs believe it or not. Here are some basic picking aids most foragers have on them whenever they're out there;

Scissors

While there is no denying that many plants can be picked easily by hand without any real effort, there are other plants that require more finesse. With some plants, you can easily twist and break while others either require way more fight or just don't yield, and even if they do, you've probably done damage to the loot or the source. Sometimes, newbie foragers pick the entire branch while trying to pick fruit. Foraging is slowly becoming a thing now, so you can easily find tools specifically for the purpose or make do with basic farming equipment. Foraging scissors are now hitting the shelves in different towns. These scissors can easily fit in your back pocket and be used for pruning and clipping different plants and fruits. Another major benefit of using scissors is that you can reach the lower ends of plants and cut them, so you have the roots intact. This way, you have a win-win situation in which you have something to eat, and you can always come back for more in the future.

Gardening Gloves

You cannot use a pair of scissors for everything. More importantly, health and safety is something no forager should ever take for granted. It's easy to convince yourself that it's just dirt, but this dirt can do unwanted to your skin. This is because bacterial and fungal infections can easily be acquired while foraging in the forest or even in your back garden. The soil in gardens is full of micro-organisms that can cause different infections along with animal droppings as well. Even though washing your hands properly should do the trick, why risk paying for all that medicine to fight off the infection when you can spend a buck or two on gloves. After all, the best medicine is prevention.

Knife

Like scissors, knives are among the basic tools every forager is known to carry. In fact, many prefer to carry knives instead of scissors. Knives come in handy for the purpose of cutting, peeling, and slicing. As any forager, and they'd have a fungus or mushroom knife in their arsenal. Even a pocket knife can be handy outdoors, especially even though it is not exactly razor-sharp. As we read, we will discuss in detail a forager's knife.

Long Sticks

Foragers usually like to pick fruit more than other things that are often found in high trees. Now, not everyone can climb a tree, which is where a long stick comes in. Now, there's not much science to how long it should be or a store that sells them. You can easily find one outdoors in the woods and use it to shake long branches to release fruits or nuts.

Hard Plastic

Shopping bags and gloves won't protect you from thorns. All gloves do is offer protection from bacteria and possibly toxic materials in the soil, but thorns will still poke you right through. If you cut up a soda bottle and use the hole to avoid thorns, you can save yourself a lot of trouble. You can even wrap prickly pears in a cardboard or a wrapping sheet to save your hands.

Ax

If you live in Alaska or anywhere in the countryside, owning an ax is pretty common. They are excellent for chopping wood and plants with strong roots. Plus, you can even find mini-axes which are much easier to carry and keep in the back of your truck or backpack.

Mini Hand Trowel

If you know your plants, you will definitely come across foraging a lot of them from their roots. There's nothing wrong with getting your hands dirty, but if you want to do things faster, a trowel is just what you need. Plus, most trowels are on the sharp side so you can use them to cut or soft roots or branches.

First Aid

It's never a bad idea to be prepared when in nature. Despite precautions, accidents can happen, and it's inevitable that you may get small injuries or even big ones. A smart forager always packs a first aid kit with basic over the counter pills and dressings. This way, they can avoid having to rush to the emergency room when they're in the middle of nowhere and also stop wounds from getting infected in time. Here are some basic first aid kit items foragers carry with them;

Band-Aids

Band-aids are basic items found in every first aid kid. Foragers often get splinters or even fall down every now and then outdoors so these can help close the wound once you've cleaned it. Plus, the band-aids also prevent further contact with the wound, so you don't get an infection.

Tweezers

Tweezers are commonly used by foragers to remove splinters and thorns. These are the most commonly occurring foraging injuries that usually people take for granted. There's always a chance that a friend might carry band-aids, but hardly anyone carries tweezers. Even if they do, it's a bad idea to share them since you know, germs.

Alcohol and Antiseptic Wipes

An Alcohol wipe is another basic item found in almost all first aid kids. They are quite helpful in preventing infections on cuts and bruises. Antiseptic wipes do the same job but don't sting like alcohol, so it's really up to you to choose what to keep.

Plantain Leaves

Any good forager knows that nature is full of medicinal plants and herbs. Plantain leaves naturally heal stings from poison ivy rashes, mosquito bites, and sunburn. However, this isn't something you'd easily find in your pharmacy or food store but can easily be another item you can forage them from yards and gardens near you. They are found almost everywhere in North America, so you should easily come across this plant when you're outdoors.

Clean Up

No matter how hard you try, there is no way you're coming back from foraging the way you left. Nature is beautiful but messy, and when foraging, you're bound to come in contact with dirt and plants along with everything else nature has to offer. So, if you have a backpack, you might want to have the following;

Water

You cannot go foraging without water. You need to keep yourself hydrated at all times as foraging can be a quite refreshing but physically exhausting experience. Plus, you're bound to get dirty and might not always be close to a water source like a lake or river nearby. So, you should always keep a water bottle with you at all times. You can also use the water to wash the plants as well before taking them home, so they are relatively clean. You never know what animal has peed on the mushrooms you just picked up or worse.

Washcloth or Tissue

You will be dealing with dirt when you're foraging, so your hands will definitely get dirty. A washcloth comes in handy when cleaning up fruits or nuts you pick up from the dirt, and wet wipes help clean you up when you're done. Plus, you can easily keep them in your back pocket or backpack.

Additional Items

While there somethings that are absolutely necessary, there way more things you can take on a foraging expedition. You can have an all-out camping trip with foraging as part of the experience, so there's no limit to what you can do. However, there are some items we feel should every forager should have with them;

Digital Camera

Foraging is a memorable experience, and for new foragers, taking pictures in the wild takes your memories home with you to show your friends and family. Plus, you can take pictures of plants you're not really sure about and check on the internet if they're edible or not.

Bear Bells

If you live in North America, especially Alaska, there are chances you might run into a grizzly passing by. Bear bells are small balls foragers tie up to their boots or stick. Their working principle is quite simple. Since there is no noise similar to bells in the forest and bears almost always want to avoid humans, they turn in the opposite direction when they hear them.

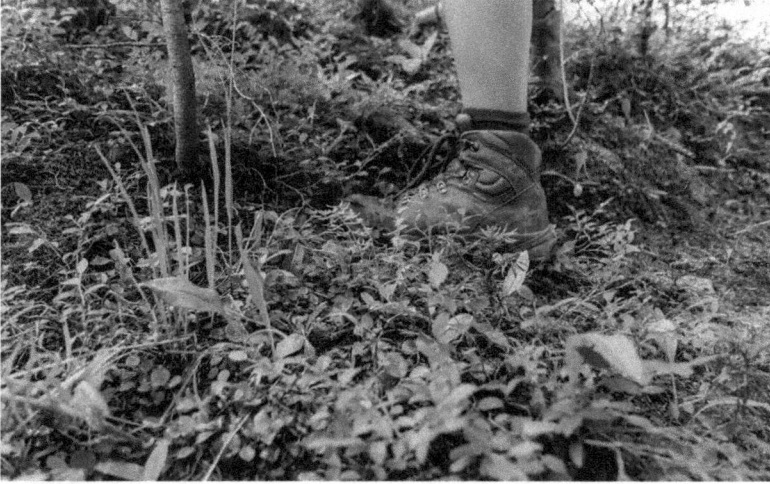

Hiking Shoes

Any joggers or running shoes would do perfectly fine, but hiking boots are a much better option for foragers. They protect your feet from rocks and debris on the ground and have a much better grip than a regular ship. They are extremely durable and suitable for outdoor activities as well as both wet and dry conditions. Moreover, they also offer protection from wild animals, especially snakes that may be hiding near the plants you're looking to pick from.

Raincoat

Foragers keep a keen eye on the weather since they'll be spending quite a bit of time outdoors. Raincoats protect you from the rain the same way as umbrellas but are much easier to handle since you'll be putting it on without carrying any real weight. So, let's say you're in the woods and it's about to pour, you can simply put on the coat to stay dry and avoid getting cold.

DIY Spice Kit

In many cases, foraging is usually part of a camping trip that involves cooking different meals. So, foragers often carry a spice kit with them, which they can fill from their homes or get from foraged items.

Torch

Depending on where you live or what time you decide to go foraging, chances are it may get dark or foggy even, so carrying a torch with you will definitely help. You can even get one in so many different shapes and sizes easily available at any hardware or convenience store.

Lighter

On many occasions, foragers look to make a meal as soon as they are done foraging. While there is nothing like going completely old school trying to make fire, there is also no shame in carrying a lighter to start a fire instantly.

A Foragers Best Friend "The Mushroom Knife"

Every forager knows that there isn't much science to collecting wild mushrooms in terms of equipment. Almost any knife will do the job but not exactly the way it should be done. You can tell a lot about a forager by their taste in knives. A mushroom knife, as the name suggests, is a knife that is specifically designed for use by mushroom enthusiasts. Like any knife, it will cut just about anything, but it is made especially for this purpose. So much so, that there are a lot of considerations that are actually put into the design. Mushrooms usually tear easily, so anyone can easily pull them from their substrate easily. The problem is that the tear can be uneven, thereby damaging either the mushroom or the mycelim it was growing on. A lot of people ask why not use a normal knife? Many foragers say that it's all about the steal as it offers a much cleaner cut. However, there are a lot more considerations put into this such as;

Safety

Any knife could slip and cut the user. Cheap folding knives without any safety lock could damage fingers upon closing. Sure, there are better folding options in the market, but that isn't the only consideration to take. What you need is something steady with a strong and steady grip.

Convenience

A forager doesn't want to be seen around holding something that looks like a machete, nor does he want to spend time looking for "Needle" in his backpack and end up cutting themselves. A foraging knife should be just the right size to be able to carry anywhere without frightening people who may find it dangerously odd looking. A small folding knife does a good job being discrete and easily goes into your pocket as well.

Durability

If you're spending a decent any money on a special knife, it has to be durable; otherwise, no one is going to buy it. The go-to option when picking a durable knife is one that is made out of stainless steel and has a strong wooden or fiber handle. You can also pick carbon fiber blades that are more expensive but much easier to sharpen than ordinary knives. Most importantly, these knives should be able to survive different conditions such as dampness, should be rust and dustproof, and light-weight.

Utility

Any knife will work on most mushrooms. However, there are some species out there that are much tougher for a regular knife to handle. Plus, just because it's called a mushroom knife does not mean that it's not going to cut anything else. The Mushroom knife you choose must work as a high-quality multi-tool with a strong blade. One thing most Mushroom knives have in common is that the blades are smaller but fatter than regular knives, which allow for a much better grip and smoother cut.

Cost

Of course, there is no consideration without looking at the cost. Any knife which isn't a regular knife would carry a higher price. There is no denying that a Mushroom knife is are quite expensive. So, unless it's going to serve a purpose, an ordinary knife cannot, there is no point in buying one unless it's just another collector's item.

After spending a decent amount of money on a knife, you should definitely learn to take care of it properly. Any good knife requires regular and proper sharpening, especially new ones, which are usually shipped out dull due to safety reasons. Even knife sharpening is a skill foragers have to learn and practice to avoid accidents or damage to the knife. Any experienced forager would tell you that you must clean your knife and fully dry it after each use. This way, it will last a bit longer and look clean as well. After all, it's not a butchering knife. There are a lot of ways to keep a knife clean and sharp for your next trip. Some people usually get a whetstone while others simply find some mineral oil to clean it with which kills two birds with one stone. Home chefs that like to cook meat at home usually have a honing rod instead of a whetstone since it is relatively easier to use.

A Forager's Skillset

Foraging is a skill on its own, and there are some pre-requisite skills that even entry-level foragers must possess if they hope to become any good at it. It's safe to say that any skill that makes you more self-sufficient easily counts in your hopes to become a forager. This includes basic survival skills, cooking, how to start a fire, growing your own food, and so much more. Apart from a list of skills that you learn over time, a forager should be an outdoor person. If you're not an outdoor person, it is very unlikely that they would make a good forager. Here are some basic things you should know or skillsets you should learn at least at a basic level;

Botany 101

There are nearly 400,000 different types of plants in the world today. So, if you are looking to become a forager, you should be able to identify plants that grow in the wild. Moreover, you should be able to distinguish between plants that look alike and know what to find near you in different seasons. You can easily find anything on the internet these days if you know what to look for. With the right approach, you'll be surprised how quickly you can start learning not only about plants but where to find them, safely extract them and even grow some at home or in your garden. In addition to all this, there are plants that are extremely dangerous to consume, so you need to be able to identify those as well. There are some signs all plants have on them, indicating if they are safe to eat or not. Obviously, there is no sure way, but experienced foragers say to stay away from plants that have a colored sap, any sort of spines, thorns or hairs, plants with bitter or soapy taste, plants with three-leaved growth patterns and seeds inside pods. Of course, there are many edible plants that show the same characteristics, but if you learn about some of them, you should have no problem finding and consuming them. Not all plants are edible but may serve well as medicine. Here are some common wild plants you should definitely be able to identify, extract and use according to its best fit;

Plantain

Plantain is a weed that will grow just about anywhere, from gardens and driveways to forests and parks in the country. You can easily pick the leaves and leave behind the stems. Plantain is used in a variety of dishes, including 5-minutes snacks in the form of chips. They are said to be gluten-free, which makes them even healthier alternative to potatoes.

Prickly Pear Cactus

Don't let looks deceive you. Prickly pears are not only edible but are packed with vitamins that provide excellent nutrition. You can easily cut off the spines and leaves then cook up both savory dishes and dessert.

Asparagus

Asparagus is one of the most commonly used ingredients in American homes. So, you'd be thrilled to learn that they grow abundantly in all parts of North America. What makes them a bit different from Asparagus you purchase from the supermarket is that they have a much thinner stalk. Plus, they're extremely easy to harvest. All you have to do is bend, twist, and snap. You can take enough for a one or two-time meal without killing the plant so you can always come back for more.

Wild Spinach

Wild spinach is better known as goosefoot. It is a fast-growing weed that can be found all over America. Most people do not cultivate them in favor of their commercially known counterparts, which makes them easily available for the taking. They are packed with nutrition, and you couldn't tell the difference from regular spinach.

Green Seaweed

Not all plants you eat come from the land. Foragers who live in coastal areas love to collect green seaweed, which is found in all the oceans of the world. You can add them to soup, rice dishes, and even make sushi at home without having to purchase expensive ingredients from the store.

Natural Medicine

Not all plants you find in the wild are edible, but this doesn't mean they are not useful. Plants also make an excellent source of natural medicine; our ancestors used thousands of years ago since there weren't any pharmacies for obvious reasons. You can find different medicinal herbs, roots, leaves, and sap for different remedies. Here are some common plants that every forager should keep an eye out for when they're outdoors;

Chamomile

Chamomile is considered to be a natural cure-all. It is commonly found in green tea and quite popular in the US as a sedative for anxiety and relaxation. So, after a long day of foraging, you can make a hot meal with chamomile tea to relax those muscles as well as your mind. However, it should not be taken in high amounts, and if you're allergic, you should avoid them.

Valerian

Valerian is found in different parts of the US and is used to treat insomnia and reduce anxiety. It is also used to flavor a variety of drinks like root beer as well as deserts. However, you should talk with your doctor before taking it as with any other medicinal herb or root.

Aloe Vera

Aloe Vera has been used for hundreds of years to treat burns, cuts, and infections. They also help with digestion and are often mixed with different oils for better hair growth. Plus, it is very easy to recognize once you know what it looks like since it doesn't really have any close relatives that look like it.

Lavender

Lavender has been used for thousands of years for its anti-inflammatory and antiseptic properties. Moreover, people are more attracted to its fragrance, which is said to help with migraine, anxiety, depression, and amnesia.

Willow Bark

Willow Bark is found all across North America and has been used for centuries as a natural pain reliever. Foragers call it nature's aspirin and often try to get their hands on it whenever they're out there.

Scout Craft

Not all foragers are boy scouts, but it's safe to say that boy scouts would definitely make great foragers. Scout craft is a modern term used to cover a variety of outdoor knowledge and skills required by people who normally seek venture into the wild country and try to sustain themselves to become more independent. This knowledge and skills are used to encourage self-reliance, resourcefulness, and confidence not just to survive but also make the best use of the natural environment around them. These skills include cooking, camp preparation, clean up, edible wild plants, fire building, first aid, hiking, knowing herbs and trees, preparing firewood, hunting, swimming, and wildlife. Scout craft is a lighter version of bushcraft, which includes tracking, hunting, fishing, shelter-building, and navigation with the use of tools such as axes, knives, foraging, wood, and natural materials. Foragers that have even some of these skills can have a much easier time in the woods to gather, transport, prepare, and consume different wild plants and fruits.

Cooking

If you're looking to become a forager, the chances are that you know your way around the kitchen. Most people have a difficult time using regular ingredients, let alone foraged ones. One of the most important benefits of cooking is that you get to control the ingredients that go into your food. Besides, one of the main ideas of foraging is to make you self-sufficient, so you don't rely on buying food all the time. This means that you cook yourself with ingredients that not a lot of people regularly use. Many foragers say that cooking a hot meal from foraged items is extremely rewarding as it means a job well done after a long od gathering and transporting wild ingredients. If you don't know how to cook, you can easily start off by making simple things like plantain chips or pan steak and season with foraged herbs and spices. Once you get the basics down, you'll become even more creative and try out more challenging foods. For instance, some foragers like to make their own root beer, pickles, and sauces ready to go at all times. With so many flavors to pick from, there's no limit to what you can do.

Foraging in the 21st Century

Foraging is a wonderful activity that connects you with nature. However, a good foraging adventure doesn't mean it should be done like our ancestors with limited tools and technology. While there's nothing wrong with doing things the old fashioned way, humans have always tried making everything they do better with the aid of technology, and the same can be said for foraging. Why go in blind when you can simply look up what you need and know exactly where to find it without too much hassle. Suppose you're on the hunt for mushrooms. You can easily search online for different species available in your area and also take some pictures with you, so when you run into one, you can check if that's what you need. Besides, it's not going to really take away the adventure since technology is always optional, and many foragers usually try to limit using gadgets in the wild. Even if they do use technology, they'll still be outdoors doing what every forager does. Using gadgets might just make things easier, but you'd still have to do them. For example, when people go camping, building a fire is one of the most important activities. However, this doesn't mean that you pick up a stick and stone and go at it for hours. There's no shame in carrying a lighter that can do the job in no time. The same way, modern foragers have the luxury to be way more tech-savvy when outdoors. Here are a few tech gadgets most foragers keep with them at all times;

A Smartphone

Most people now own a smartphone and take it with them wherever they go. So, why should foraging be any different? As long as you have cellular reception, you can easily search for anything on the internet in the middle of a forest or park. If you come across a plant that you're not sure of, you can take a picture and ask your peers to confirm. A smartphone is practically a computer in your pocket, so the use cases are endless when it comes to research. Plus, most smartphones have compasses and maps in them, so you don't need to carry either to save room for more loot.

Camping Cookware

Camping cookware usually consists of pans, pots, cutlery, and utensils, along with food containers that are specifically built for the outdoors. You can imagine why most foragers would like to get their hands on some of these items. As mentioned earlier, many foragers have admitted that most of their adventures involved foraging, but foraging wasn't the sole purpose of the trip. Many foragers love camping with their friends and family, and this is where cookware comes in extremely handy for them. However, for those who carry cookware on their foraging venture, it is usually to prepare a meal outside rather than transporting it home.

Multi-Toolkit

Foragers love to accessorize with gadgets that could make their venture easier. A multi-toolkit that fits into your pocket with different functions like altimeter, barometer, thermometer, LED light, and different blades can come in extremely handy during the search and extraction of different plants and fruits.

Digital Binoculars

Binoculars were among the few gadgets outdoor enthusiasts always wanted even as kids. To be able to look into the distance and explore nature with a closer view is extremely satisfying. From a forager's perspective, being able to spot berries and fruits high up in trees from a distance can help pick them much quicker and also be on a lookout since the woods are no short of wild animals that can cause harm up close. Today, you can even find digital binoculars than offer functions like digital zoom and video recording so you can always go back and not only relive your adventure but also share with others as well.

Foraging Guidelines to Remember

For those who are really keen on becoming a forager or just looking at it as a hobby to pass the time, these are just some of the things you can do or learn to become better each and every day. Like we mentioned earlier, foraging is a patience game since you cannot always plan ahead, nor will you always return with something. Even with all the technology we have today, you still have to learn the basics if you really want to adapt to life. You can start off by deciding what kind of forager you are hoping to become. People have different reasons for getting started. Some say they would like to save money while others have their own land so they can not only grow their own food but also forage what's readily available. Outdoor enthusiasts can add to their list of possible recreational activities, while those who love to cook can add unique flavors to their everyday menu with foraged items. Whatever your reasons are, these guidelines will definitely help you;

Be Safe

It is important that you do not take safety for granted. Make sure that you are 100 percent sure in your identification of wild plants so you don't consume anything that may harm you. Always carry a basic first aid kit, water, a few snacks, and be aware of where you are. Before you harvest, have a good look at the plant for any wildlife and also any signs that may say private property or no trespassing. Try to avoid those areas where you know plants may have been exposed to toxins like near factories or commercial areas.

Be Respectful

A lot of foragers have been arrested in the past for unintentionally trespassing property. If you're looking to go on a foraging venture, you should know who's land you'll be on and get permission first. National parks are off-limits as well as public places. Usually, you will see no-picking signs if foraging isn't allowed. Apart from the rules, be respectful to the plants as well. If you dig up holes, make sure you fill it back. Also, don't damage or kill the plant just for a free meal and definitely don't let foraged food go to waste.

Be Sustainable

Invasive species of plants are fair game all year round so you can throw a buffet party if it pleases you. However, most plants require more attention, so you need to look up their growth patterns and only harvest them at the optimum time. Otherwise, the plant may not taste really good, and you would have wasted its growth for the season.

Learn In Person

There is a lot to learn when it comes to foraging. The best way to learn is from another forager or taking a class. This way, you can learn it properly in an organized manner without any distractions and complete attention to the details. You can also visit a local herbalist to learn more about what you can find in your area. If you're simply looking for a hobby to kill time, there is sufficient information on the internet, and in this book, as you read further, you could use to find something for your next meal. All you'd need is a good pair of shoes, a backpack, smartphones, and something to cut like a pair of scissors or a pocket knife.

Chapter 5

Foraging for Food

It is no big secret that our generation is not equipped with foraging knowledge and skills as extensively as our hunter-gather ancestors. As a successful forager, it is imperative to identify the wild plants, seeds, and nuts –harmful or safe– with no possibility of error. An enthusiastic forager may be excited to learn all about the bounty nature offers, but wandering out to the nearest field to handpick and eat random plants is a recipe for disaster. Naturally, newcomers may want to try everything they come across; however, such practice can be a massive risk to their lives. Although some wild plants may only cause minor health issues, for example, a stomachache, many might be poisonous, resulting in something much worse.

For over 25 years, Green Deane, a famous foraging YouTuber, has gained expertise in a vast majority of North America's plants growing in the wild. According to him, only 7% of wild plants are edible; this stresses how essential it is to be able to identify various plants, seeds, and nuts that can be eaten, but more importantly, which should be avoided. To help out amateurs, Deane has outlined four major steps every forager must remember to confirm the edibility of any wild plant by using a system known as "ITEM"; Identification, Time of the year, Environment, and Method of preparation.

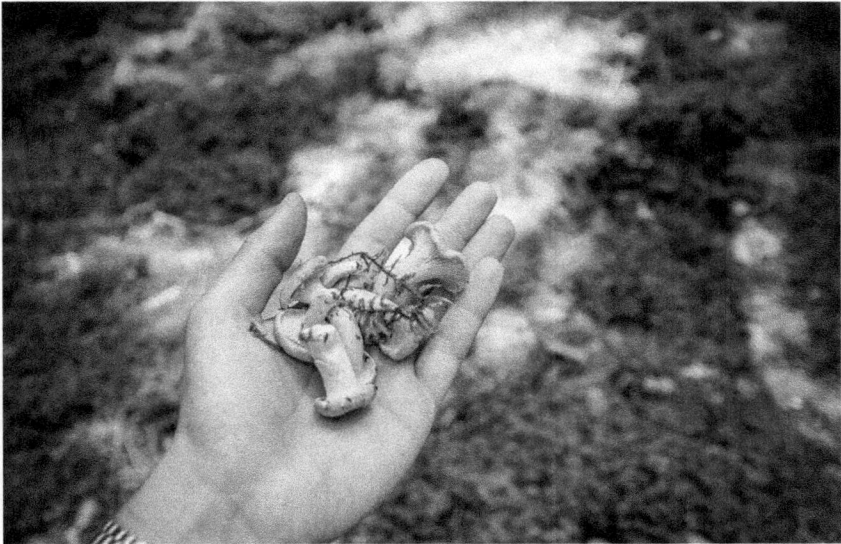

Identification

It is crucial for both amateurs and experts to identify plants correctly and to know if it is edible, beyond all possibility of doubt. Newcomers must receive a pass from a local foraging expert before they swallow anything they have handpicked. It is dangerous to depend on pictures from guidebooks and the internet for this activity –different plants look different in varying climates and environments. They might even have lethal lookalikes, proving it necessary to consult someone who knows how a certain plant looks like in their area. Over time, people would be able to indulge in foraging independently as they master the skills and knowledge of their territories, but even then, they should practice caution.

Time of Year

Due to phenology, climate, or the growth stage of the plant, the same plant species experience differing qualities throughout the year. The forage quality of a plant may vary even during the same months in different years. Such factors make the whole identification process trickier; hence, foragers need to recognize if a plant is growing, or producing vegetables or fruit, at the appropriate time of the year. If a flower is known for blooming in March, but it is found sprouting in September, it is highly probable that it is a close relative, maybe a non-edible one. Additionally, this might also indicate a gap in the forager's knowledge. For example, Pyracantha coccinea is a firethorn bush, known to bloom and bear fruit once a year in northern regions; however, it was also discovered in Florida where it blooms twice a year in two different seasons. This is why if foragers come across plant species exhibiting differing qualities than what they are usually known for, they should consult an expert.

Environment

Some would say it is more important, and often trickier, to identify the plant's environment than the plant itself. A forager should confirm that the soil and water surrounding it are not polluted, mixed with gasoline or other chemicals. Plants growing in various areas like someone's garden, a field, city parks, etc. could have been treated with pesticides. All of these environmental factors could make them unsafe to eat, which contributes more to the reason why people should thoroughly inspect what they eat.

Another reason to be environment-conscious is that plants have particular soil, water, temperature, and sunlight preferences; this makes the whole identification process easier if the forager is well-equipped with such knowledge, and can readily identify the plant himself.

Method of Preparation

Foragers may come across multiple plants classified as edible; however, it does not necessarily mean they are ready-to-eat. Many wild plants need to be soaked in salty water, cooked, peeled, etc. before they can be eaten. Therefore, knowing what it takes to make the wild plant edible is also an essential aspect before it is consumed.

This method has helped out thousands to forage safely. However, it only reduces a handful of risks that accompany this activity –not eradicate them. Although the plant itself is edible, it may trigger the person's food intolerance or allergies. Especially while trying out new plants, foragers should expose themselves to one new plant at a time, so if they have any unanticipated reactions later, they would precisely know what caused it.

The first wise thing to do is to rub the plant against one's skin to see if it develops a rash. If all is well, the next step is to rub it against lips and wait before taking a bite. Deane recommends taking only a few bites when trying out a new wild plant. Even then, the first successful trial run sometimes does not guarantee that a person will not develop a rash later. Thus, an individual should limit himself to small portions before he feels confident enough to make it a regular part of his diet.

As stressed multiple times before, you should never put something in your mouth if you are not 100% sure if it is edible. To make the foraging process easier for everyone, a list of most commonly found wild fruits, nuts, and seeds in North America has been prepared. Some of these might be rare, while others are popular and even cultivated on a large scale. Additionally, pictures have also been added to aid the identification of wild plants with easy techniques and simple descriptions. Enclosed with them, you will find the tasty edible's key characteristics, usage, as well as their harvesting time and method, included below.

Chapter 6

Guide to Identifying Editable Fruits

American Crabapples

A particular specie of crabapples, Malus Coronaria, is a native to North America. It goes by the name American crabapples, sweet crabapples, etc. Overall, around 30 species of crabapples exist, among which several of them are scattered around the continents, exceptionally hardy in 4 to 8 USDA zones. It has many hybrid species; therefore, its identification can be tricky.

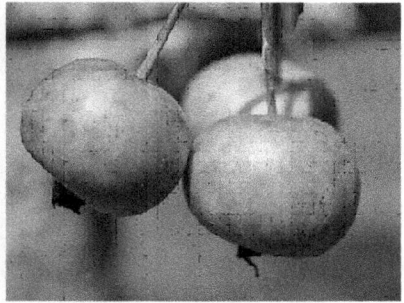

The American crabapple's tree can grow from 5 to 30 feet in height, with a wide-open crown, stout branches, and a short trunk. Its leaves are alternate, teethed edges, a heart-shaped or round base, and usually narrow long-pointed tips. Moreover, its bark is greyish-brown and scaly, making it easy for it to peel off. The flowers start blooming on the American Crab in spring, which is highly fragranced and colored either white or pink. They might be small in size but bountiful. The trees bear fruits from September to November, which are green-yellow, bitter, and several-seeded. Due to their citric acid and malic content, they can be tannic or very sour, and so, not consumed raw very often. Instead, they are roasted first before being devoured or used to make home-made country wine or cider, etc.

American Cranberry

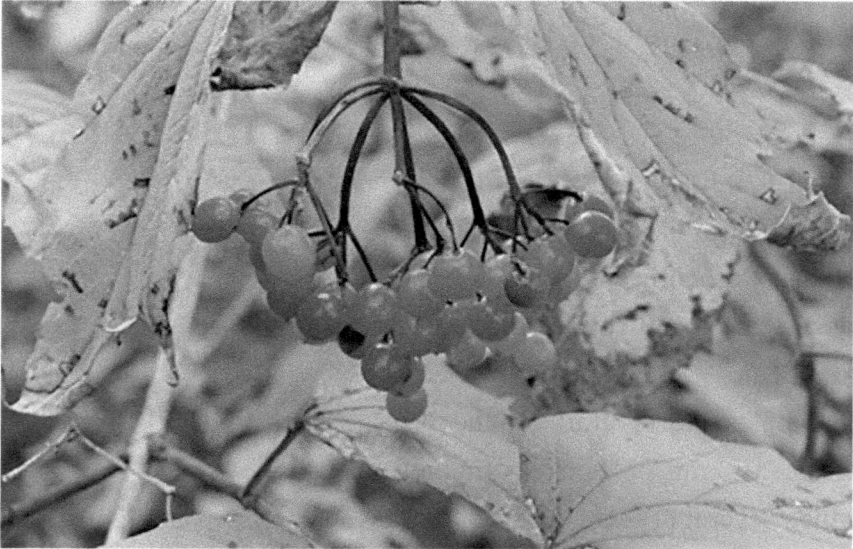

The American cranberry bush, although native to South America, is a rare find. The shrub is found scattered in areas north of Illinois, and other high-quality wetlands with native flora being still intact. Its habitats are various, with it being spotted in sandy swamps, forested bogs, soggy thickets, roadside ditches, moist woodlands, streambanks of wooded areas, etc. It helps if the ground has decaying organic matter as it helps retain moisture. Furthermore, the bush prefers to grow in full sun (and sometimes light shade too), and a boreal climate where even the summers are moderately warm or cool.

To identify the American cranberry bush, one should look for multiple narrow trunks that ascend towards arching or dense upright branches, creating a round outline. Its height together measures up to 6 to 12 feet, sometimes even shooting up to 16 feet. Its leaves also hold resemblance to maple leaves; they are a pair of opposite-growing leaves, occurring along with twigs and shoots. The foliage is deciduous, colored medium green in the upper surface and pale green on the lower. Later, during the fall, they become bright red. Furthermore, the leaves are three-lobed with slight large teeth, which sometimes are just absent altogether. The cranberry shrub bears white, 5-petaled, flat-topped clusters of flowers during late spring to early summer, lasting about approximately a whole month. When they mature during late summer or early fall, they become bright red, much like its leaves.

After they are harvested, they can be stored inside freezers and eaten later, but what most people don't know is that they can also freeze under the snow. Therefore, when the spring arrives, and the snow melts, they are still perfectly edible and can be eaten, although they might be a little soft after being thawed.

American Elderberry

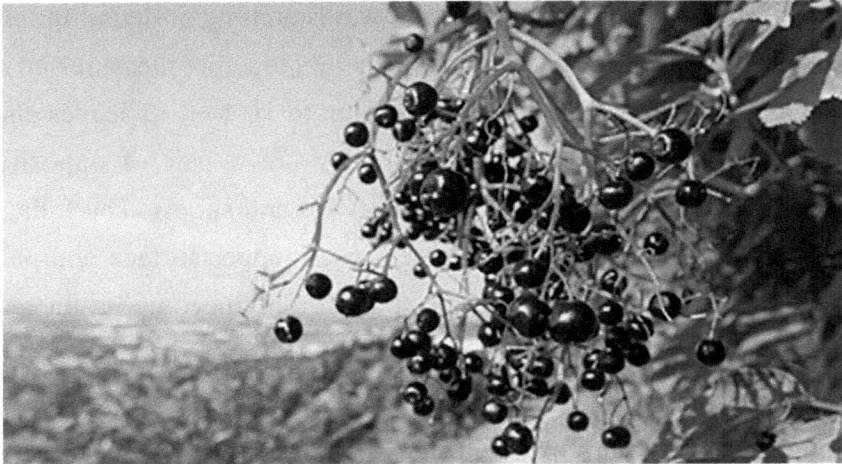

The American elderberry, also known as Sambucus Canadensis, is native to North and Central America. Tart and tangy, they should not be consumed raw, but instead sweetened to be made into elderberry syrup or tea. Too many raw elderberries, especially the under-ripe ones, can cause nausea, but boiling them in for 15 to 20 minutes takes care of that problem –if coupled with some sugar, the liquid boils to form a syrup that can be later drizzled over some yogurt or ice-cream. Cooking them inactivates their alkaloid compounds, after which they are used to make jams, juices, elderberry wine, etc. They come with their own sets of benefits; rich in vitamins A, B6, C, and other nutrients, they effectively boost the immune system and heart. It is often also taken a supplement to treat flu symptoms and cold.

Foragers often discover them on moist woodlands, fence rows, streambanks, roadsides, and thickets throughout Missouri. Although these berries are identifiable, they usually blend in with the scenery, making them hard to spot. In diameter, they are about 1/8th of an

432

inch and have a slight bump from where they sprouted from the flower. Altogether, these berries form an umbrella-shaped cluster, growing on shrubs reaching heights up to 12 feet, and sometimes even 15 feet tall.

Tiny white flowers blossom in June and July, after which deep elderberries dominate the plants in late summer. Deep purple or almost-black color indicates ripeness, which is another important factor to remember. Under-ripe elderberries, along with it red stems and leaves, can be toxic for the human body. However, its flowers can be cooked or eaten raw.

American Elderberry lookalikes:

American Pokeweed

American Pokeweed (also known as American Pokeberry, Phytolacca Americana, etc.) is one of the toxic elderberry lookalikes. Pokeweed is not edible, and should definitely be kept away from children like all other poisonous substances. They are known to cause severe stomachaches, and because its berries and red stems can be easily confused with elderberries, it is crucial to educate everyone on how to distinguish between the two.

Also native to North America, the non-woody and robust shrubs can be found almost all over the country near forest openings and edges, fences rows, pastures, etc. especially, where birds are able to roost. The plant is poisonous to touch, from the fruit to the root, and should not be touched with bare hands.

Although elderberries and pokeberries might pose strikingly similar appearances at first glance (both having dark purple-black berries), they have a few visible characteristics that help foragers to distinguish between the two. If both of these shrubs are compared, Pokeweed has shorter red stems, and the berries are firmly attached to the main stem. Moreover, this shrub grows to be a maximum of 6 feet tall, unlike its lookalike. Lastly, as their pictures indicate, elderberries grow in clusters, whereas pokeberries hang in the shape of a long cylindrical cone.

Aralia spinosa

Aralia spinosa (also known as the devil's walking stick or Hercules club) is widespread in mid-west and the eastern United States along the Atlantic coast and westward towards Texas. The chances of humans encountering these species are only high in their zones of habitation –the outer edges of temperate forests. It may often masquerade as the American berry as they also have dark purple-black berries growing on vivid burgundy stems. Both plants bear berries of similar sizes, thriving in the same kind of environment and sprouting fruits around the same time of the year. However, its berries are mildly toxic to humans, and only its leaves are ruled as edible. If the raw berries or seeds are eaten, they may cause an upset stomach.

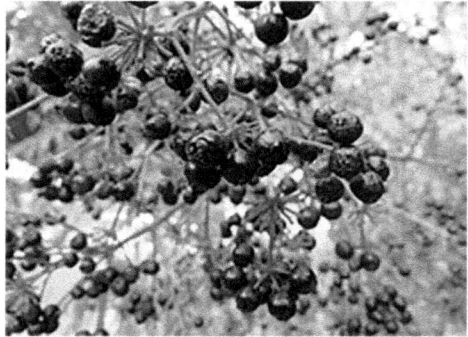

What sets them apart is their stem; Aralia's stem is thorny. The thorns can be daunting 1.25 cm long, aptly deriving the name devil's walking stick from them. On the other hand, American elders have smooth stems with limited spines and thorns. Additionally, in appearance, Aralia is a flat-topped, spiny shrub growing to a height of 25 to 35 feet typically, and may even develop as a small tree.

American Gooseberry

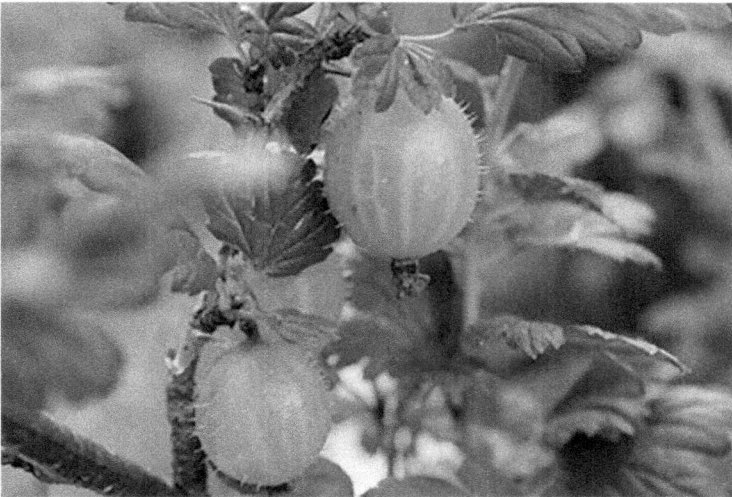

Around 100 varieties of gooseberries are growing in North America, yet people are unaware of this beauty's existence. Pop one in your mouth and you would be in for either a sour or a sweet surprise. The little treat ranges in flavor as it does in variety. It can be pretty much found everywhere in the continent except the deserts, but even then, a few species of gooseberries strive in arid regions as well. It is known to be a cold climate treat, growing in areas with warm winters and humidity as well as frosty ones.

First and foremost, to identify them, one should look for thorns on the branches, and many times, on the berries itself. These thorns are a hallmark of the gooseberry clan and a direct giveaway to the plant's existence. At every axil, the American gooseberry has two or more spines, but they are not poisonous. Some of the plant's species may bear very prickly fruits and should be harvested with gloves and necessary precautions. The second giveaway is maple-like leaves which look something like this:

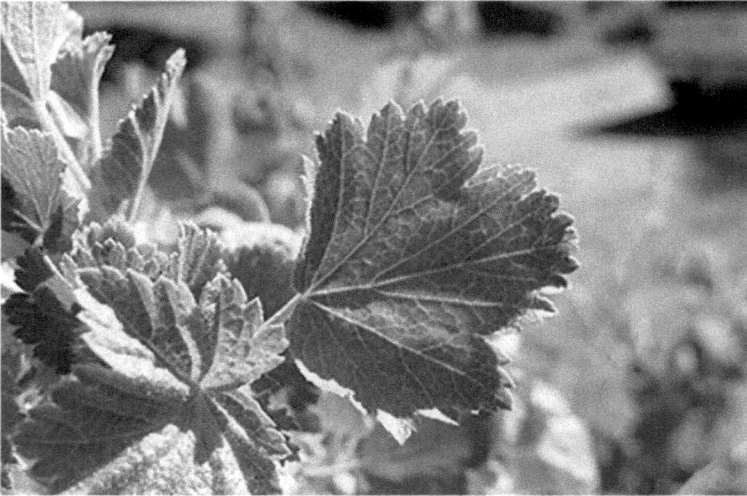

The shrub can grow 3 feet tall and 6 feet wide. The gooseberry's color and shape can vary; they are found in red, yellow, green, purple, and white colors, among which some are round, oval, or elongated. Moreover, minuscule edible seeds are also found embedded sometimes that are safe to consume like the fruit. Even if they can be eaten raw, many prefer to boil and sweeten them to use as syrups or in pies.

American Persimmon

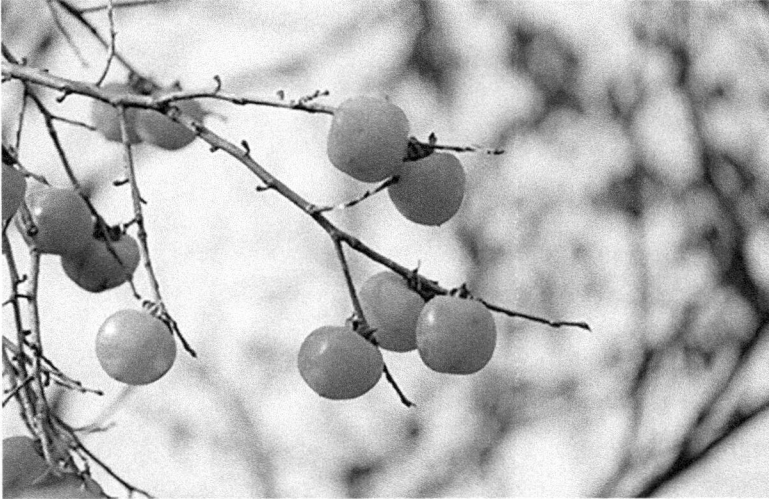

Foragers easily recognize wild American Persimmon as it is another popularly cultivated fruit, readily available at supermarkets and within people's reach. However, unlike the cultivated Asian ones, the American wild fruits are marginally smaller (much like cherry tomatoes) and the trees, prolific. They are particularly hardy to Zone 5, discovered in eastern USA's hardwood forests. These vitamins A and C-rich fruits are pulpy and sweet with a hint of spiciness. Typically, they ripen in November, so beware; they will taste bitter and astringent if they have not matured enough. Like its Asian counterpart, it can also be consumed raw, baked, or mashed.

Persimmon's bark is another distinctive feature. It's dark and forms patterns of blocks and vertical ridges that run up and down its trunk. The twigs and branches are thin, smooth, and grayish-brown in color. The fruits grow in small clusters, have flattened seeds, and are incredibly juicy. Its foliage is also alternate; they are around 2.5 to 6 inches long and ovate to elliptic-oblong in shape. The upper surface of the leave is medium to dark green and glossy, whereas, the lower one is pale green, softer, and leathery.

Black Cherry

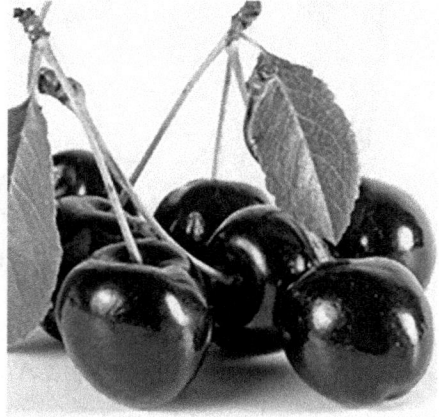

Prunus serotine (common name: Black cherry) is native to North America, Central America, and Mexico. They grow in southeastern Canada, spreading through the eastern USA and also being spotted in the mountains of the southwestern continent. The deciduous tree or shrub can grow up to 25-110 feet. It transforms from a distantly conical shape to an oval-headed one when it grows and matures, with spreading and arching branches and pendulous limbs. The foliage is glossy on the upper surface with a tapering base, blade oblong with a long-pointed tip, and finely serrated margins. When these glossy leaves emerge, the white flowers also sprout hanging in drooping racemes.

As the name indicates, the black cherry is indeed black or deep purple in color, which switches from a dark red in August through October. During the same period, the foliage also turns yellow. Cherries are consumed raw and even used to prepare jellies, wines, and other beverages because of their sweet and tart taste. Any other parts should not be tried; they are toxic due to amygdalin contained in them and may be fatal if someone accidentally ingests them. Symptoms may include spasms, convulsions, respiratory failure, pupil dilation, weakness, etc. Therefore, foragers should be extra careful not to taste them.

Although only the bearing fruits are edible, the different parts of the tree can also be put to different uses. The cherry syrup, obtained from the bark, is useful for curing coughs. On the other hand, it's wood is also very valuable, thereby, used in furniture, professional and scientific instruments, paneling, etc.

Blueberry

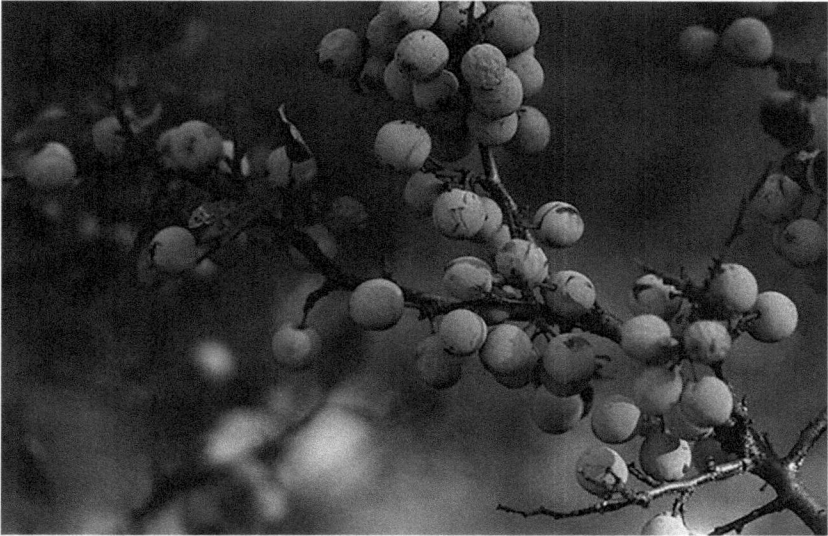

Wild blueberry plants are a low-maintenance, naturally-growing crop that produces round blue-black fruits. The plant is sub-categorized into two primary species that grow in North America – lowbush blueberry and the sour top. As their name indicates, lowbush is shorter in height (from 3 to 15 inches) and sweet, whereas sour tops are less sweet and more massive (reaching up to 24 inches tall). Where these wild blueberries can be located in North America depends on which particular specie the forager is searching for. Although they grow throughout the continent —most prevalent in New Jersey and Maine—, the sour top predominantly grows in woodlands while the lowbush is suited for forests and fields.

To identify these, one should inspect the underside of these berries. They are marked with a five-pointed crown, which is a distinct characteristic of this fruit. The branches are thin, leaves are broad and green (which later turns red in the fall season), and the flowers white and light pink in color. These wild berries are relatively smaller than cultivated blueberries -around 1/4th of an inch in diameter— but are known to be more beneficial. They are richly packed with fiber, antioxidants, and vitamin C and K.

To reap maximum benefits and excellent taste from this particular fruit, the forager needs to practice caution while harvesting them. The plants bear fruit from mid to late summer and take several days to ripe even after they turn blue. The safest approach is to tickle the blueberry bunch and eat only those who fall off without much effort.

Wild Blueberry lookalikes:

Huckleberry

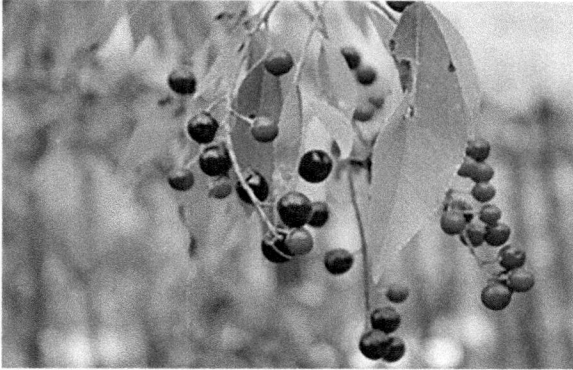

A wild shrub that is often mistaken for blueberries is Huckleberry. Although the two berries can be confused because of their similar shape and size, blueberries are a shade lighter. Even its leaves are a shade different; whereas blueberry's turn bright red in the fall, Huckleberry's leaves can turn from golden to reddish-purple. The latter's shrub is tall, growing up to whopping 4 feet (a giant compared to the lowbush blueberries) and grows faster than its lookalike. Each Huckleberry has 10 seeds, relatively harder than blueberry. An exciting aspect for both of these berries is that they can be consumed fresh, without needing to be cooked or boiled. So even if individual misidentified huckleberry, and ate it thinking it was a blueberry instead, he would be in for a tart and sweet surprise.

Present in the colors black, blue, and red, huckleberries are the North American representation of several plant species in Gaylussacia and Vaccinium genera. These small, blue wild berries grown in forests, lake basins, mountainous regions, and bogs in Western Canada and Northwestern America.

Chokeberry

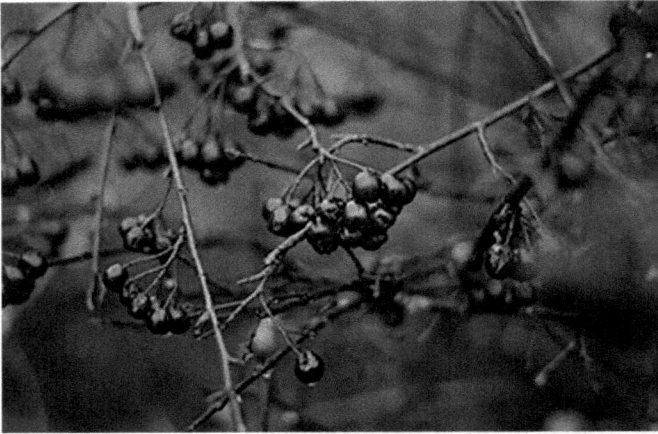

Found in Eastern Canada and Eastern America, chokeberries are a deciduous shrub, also known as Aronia. Although chokeberries are another blueberry lookalike, they are less edible wild plants. Red (Aronia arbutifolia), purple (Aronia prunifolia), and black (Aronia melanocarpa) chokeberries sprout from the plant that should be avoided from being consumed raw. The fruits are juiced, baked, or boiled before they are consumed. It is because they are highly astringent; however, they have an exceptional level of antioxidants. Having anthocyanin, proanthocyanidin, phenolic acid, and flavanol, they beat the antioxidant capacities of all other fruits. Such powerful compounds, coupled with high levels of vitamin K boost essential bodily functions and support bone health.

Typically, chokeberries feel dry to touch and have a wrinkly appearance. Regardless of the color of the fruits, they all need to be harvested as soon as they are ripe, or the risk of them drying up is high. Beautiful flowers bloom on the plants during spring, but when fall approaches, they start ripening. Blackberries are known to ripen earliest, followed by purple and then red chokeberries from mid-August to mid-September. However, they can survive in the cold, so the fruits persist long after September and make winter foraging possible. They grow in clusters of 2 to 20 berries on shrubs as tall as 8 feet, where every single fruit drops droops from its individual stem. This makes it easier to harvest wild foraged Aronia berries with fingers, quickly stripping them from their stems.

Brambles (Blackberry and Raspberry)

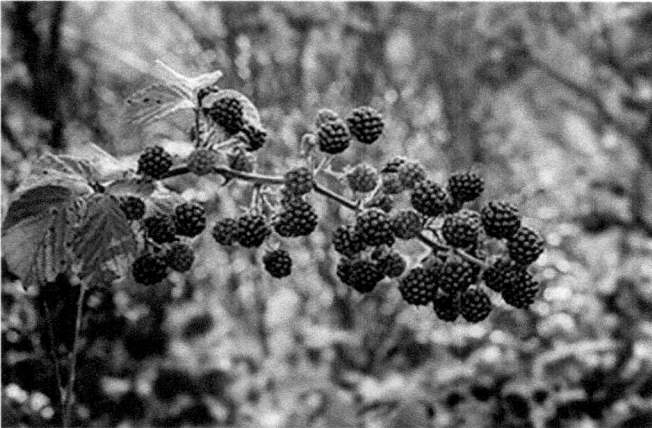

Both raspberries and blackberries identify as brambles. They may be widely cultivated throughout North America, but it's popularity also stems from their growth in the wild. Blackberries are most prevalent around the east and coastal west, whereas raspberries are pretty common all over the continent except the Deep South.

The canes on which these berries grow on are long and prickly, situated in the edges of fields and meadows under the sun. The thorny shrubs are a dead giveaway of brambles and an important factor in identifying them. They are best handled with gloves while harvesting them off their long cone-shaped clusters. Both berries ripen midsummer; typically, raspberries are either black or red when ripe, whereas, blackberries turn from green to red, and to finally black when they have ripened. Raspberries are recognized by their hollow center and round prickly stems, while on the other hand, the majority of the blackberry species curve their thick cane back to the ground; this makes them prolific as it roots once again. Moreover, their compound leaves are 5 to 25 cm long with 3 to 7 leaflets. These leaves are greatly medicinal and can be used to make tea to treat sore throats. The fruits, themselves, can be devoured raw, baked, or used in a salad (raspberries), etc.

Raspberry lookalike:

Thimbleberry

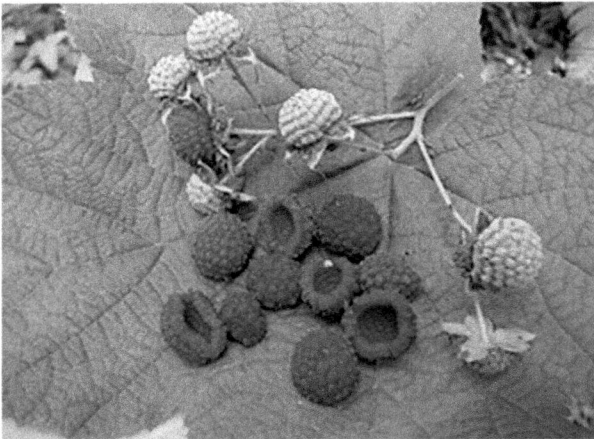

When ripe, Thimbleberries (Rubus parviflorus) maybe sometimes mistaken as Raspberries because of their deep-red colors and similar appearance. It does not pose a problem because they are delicious and completely edible lookalike. They are even known as flowering raspberries. However, on close inspection, thimbleberries are, in fact, smaller and almost hemispherical. In between, they have a hollow center, intense and incredibly flavorful taste, and are soft to touch. These berries are very soft and delicate, too, and start getting spoilt a few hours after they are harvested. Therefore, they cannot be stored for long and must be consumed soon. It is also why they can never be found at grocery stores, and it is always a treat to discover them accidentally, growing wild in woodland edges.

The fruit is native to the western and northern temperate regions of North America. The plants are large, about 6 to 8 feet in height, and approximately 3 feet in width. Its flowers may either be white or pink, depending on which species the plants belong to. Moreover, they have five flimsy petals, and their domed center is what later develops into the fruit. The fruits hang from large, thorn-less, and arching canes that are 2-3 feet tall. In proportion to the fruit, the leaves of the plants are massive (around 8 inches) and somewhat share a resemblance with maple leaves. They may even be slightly serrated or scalloped. The surrounding environment of thimbleberry plants is also a notable factor in identifying the plant. It grows around sunny patches of forests, even in areas that might have been recently disturbed by logging or fires. It is rare to find them in deep shade areas or mature forests, where sunlight does not reach.

Cloudberry

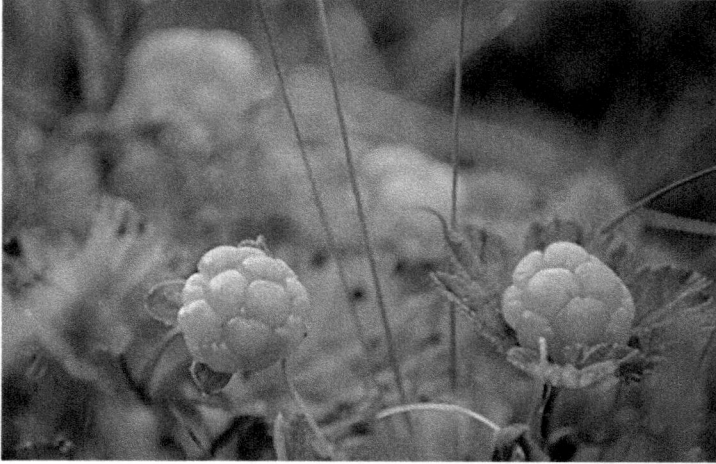

Cloudberries (Rubus chamaemorus) are widely distributed in America, especially Northern Canada and Alaska, as they prefer northern subarctic climates and boggy conditions to flourish. The plants can be both males and females in any particular area. The females may not blossom for up to 7 years, and even after they start bearing fruit, they might not necessarily produce fruit every season. They have a reasonably large seed, in proportion to the fruit itself. Each stem produces a single berry that is rich in vitamin C and contains powerful antioxidants.

They taste sweet and tart and are used as an ingredient in confections, jams, desserts, but their flavor is not what makes them stand. These rare wild berries are a beauty, with a sunny amber hue. It starts as a white, light-pinkish color, which then grows into a bright red. When it ripens, the fruit turns yellowish-orange, but some maintain their reddish tinge. Cloudberries can be consumed raw, but plucking them at the right ripening stage is the key. They are sour and crunchy if picked early, but if over-ripe, they may squish in hand at the slightest touch. Nevertheless, cloudberries are one of the exceptions that can be picked early while still unripe and will ripen up in a couple of days.

Mulberry

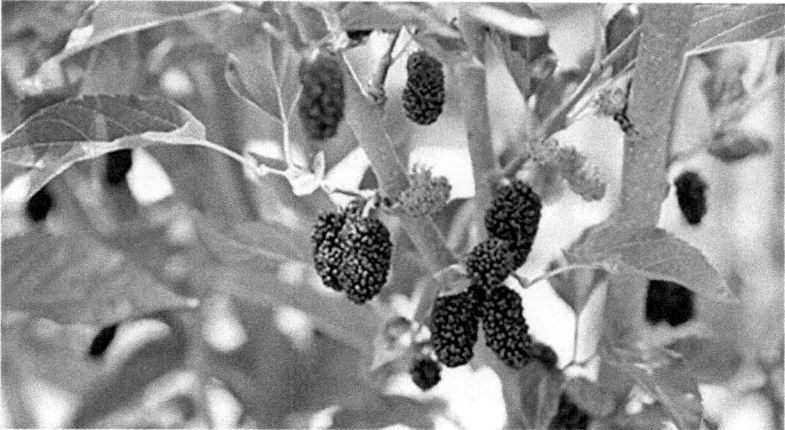

If you ever come across blackberries growing on trees, they are actually mulberries. They might resemble each other a lot, but they actually belong to the Moraceae family, with its trees rooted in the eastern United States and stretching up into Canada. These trees will usually also be near a water source. The fruit it bears is around 2 to 3 cm in length in purplish-black, red or white color typically. Unless the fruits are covering the tree, it can be a bit too tricky to identify it's a mulberry tree.

The shape of its leaves differ from specie to specie, but sometimes, even the leaves sprouting from the same branch are different. A short, heart-shaped leaf usually indicates a black mulberry tree. Rounded-teeth on the edges of the leaf means its either a red or a while mulberry tree; white leaves are relatively glossier than red mulberry leaves. Amongst the three, the black mulberry trees are the shortest; it grows 20 to 30 feet in height, white ones range from 30 to 35 feet, and the red ones are the tallest, standing more than 40 feet sometimes. Furthermore, they produce berries at different times of the year. Red mulberries, the strongest in flavor (sweetness and tartness mixed), sprout in the spring along with the white ones. They are harvested easily by shaking the tree. The black ones are mildly sweet infused with some tartness and are renowned as having the best taste, although their harvest is done in summer. They need to be handpicked as the berries cling to the branches. All of them can be eaten raw, baked, or made into wines. Up till now, there is no data on any poisonous lookalikes, so mulberries are a safe bet for those new to foraging and can be eaten without much forethought.

Muscadine

Muscadines are a grapevine species also native to the United States, most prevalent throughout Florida. They have bronze, dark purple, and black thick, leathery skin and have a texture similar to that of plums. They may be the best-tasting grapes one might come across, either on an erect vine standing tall at 90 feet or on a vine spread over small trees and low shrubs as a prostrate sprawling groundcover. When they first

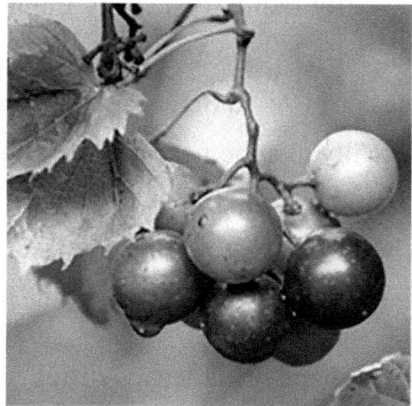

sprout from the bud, they are green but soon ripen to a blackish-purple in September to October. A musky and mildly sweet flavor is a trademark for Muscadine grapes after they are ripe and have dropped to the ground.

To identify this specie, one should pay attention to their foliage. The leaves are satin, dark green on top and yellow on the underside, or vice versa (especially in fall). They reveal no lobes and have smaller leaves and fruits, relative to other grape species. They also have deeply serrated and coarse edges in the shape of a heart. The fruits are loosely arranged in small clusters, and the bark is gray-brown, smooth, and non-peeling, unlike other grape species in gardens.

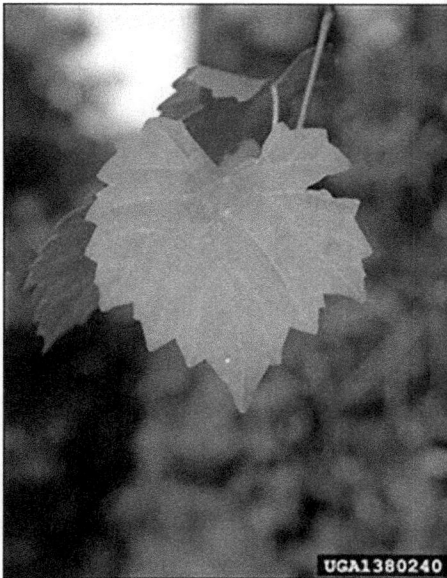

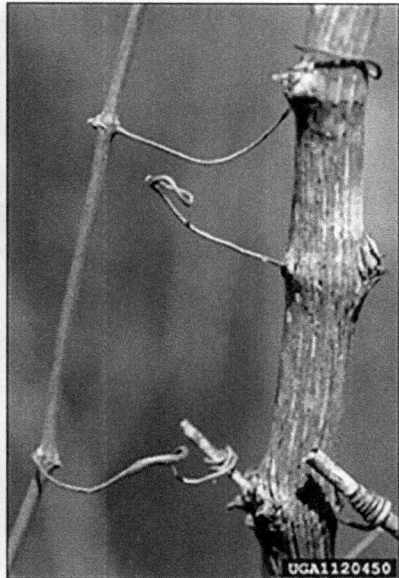

Pawpaws

Pawpaws are tropical, mango-like fruits, mostly accessible to individuals who handpick them from trees. It is renowned as the largest North American fruit, with homely and speckled skin, and a custard-like texture that tastes delicate and delicious. Its taste is said to range somewhere between a mango and banana, although some people swore to have sensed a hint of pineapples, melon, and other fruitarian delicacies. It's safe to say the flavor differs from tree to tree. It can be eaten raw, the sweet flesh directly scooped out into a ball, and the seeds separated. Pawpaw's seeds are toxic, and therefore, you should not eat the fruit directly. The fruit starts ripening from late August to October; pawpaws fall from their trees when fully ripe but can be shaken from their branches when they are close to being fully ripened.

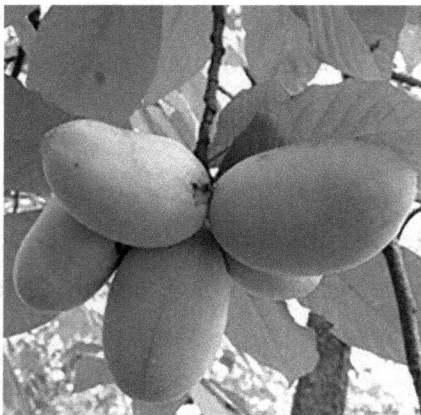

Wild pawpaws are common in eastern America, usually growing alongside riverbanks. The dense thicket trees can be found growing in northern Florida to southern Ontario, and even touches the west (Texas), hidden under the shade of surrounding taller trees. This edible wild fruit indigenous to North America has a few species among which some have dwarf trees (around 4 to 5 feet) while others sprout up to 40 feet tall. Its leaves are alternate, smooth and can be as big as 20 inches.

Saskatoon Berries

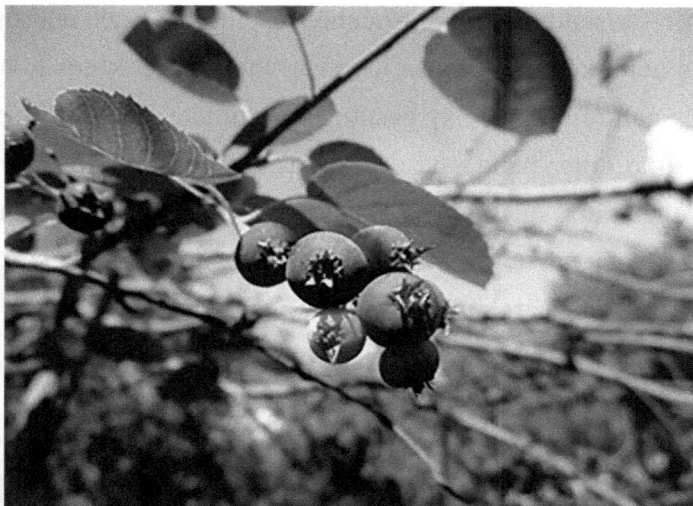

Saskatoon berries also commonly go by Juneberries, Serviceberries, and Shadbush, divided into many different species growing in various regions of Canada and the United States. Some are found growing along the East Coast, while others are prevalent in the pacific northwest. They are a deep purple-blue when fully ripe; otherwise, a pinkish tinge is present. They taste delicious and have said to transcend over all other wild berries with its sweet flavor. Not everyone is lucky enough to come across these berries growing in the wild, though; the birds strip them off the plants when they have just begun to turn pink in late June or early July. Depending on the species, Saskatoon shrubs can grow from 3 to 26 feet. Because some of them are very tall and out of arm's reach, the birds get to them first. Typically, these sought-after annual treats can be found near hillsides, riverbanks, along roadsides, and in woods.

These plants cannot survive in heavy clay or poorly drained soils at all and prefer sandy loam. Serviceberries' resemblance and the taste is very much like blueberries; however, their larger seeds give away their true nature. Each berry has an approximate diameter of 5 to 15 mm. On the other hand, the deciduous leaves are 3 to 6 cm long, oblong and round at the base. They will have soft, fine hair when they are not mature, but will be smooth, similarly like its twigs. Often, its branches arch upwards to be parallel with the main stem.

Strawberry

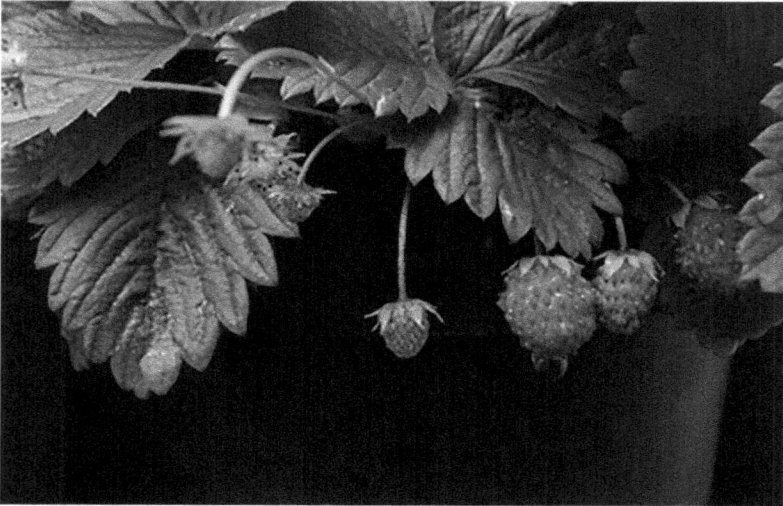

Although strawberries are widely cultivated in America and present at every grocery store, they cannot rival the burst of flavor its wild version contains. Wild strawberries (Fragaria Virginiana) might be a tad smaller than their commercial cousins, but full of flavor. Some foragers have pointed out how these berries emit such a sweet and powerful aroma that they smell the fruit way before they spot them.

The wild strawberry plants are easily identifiable through their five-petal white flower and cluster of three jagged leaves with hairy undersides, even if the fruits have not sprouted yet. The white flower has a yellow center, which then later changes into a delicate fruit.

The wild strawberry plants are popular all over America except Hawaii, growing to a height of 5 to 15 cm tall. It starts developing in early spring and looks pretty much like cultivated strawberries with tiny-seed like appearance on its skin. However, they also produce long, dull red-colored hairy runners through which they reproduce, forming plantlets. Almost all parts of the wild strawberry plant –the fruit, flower, and leaves– are edible and used for multiple purposes.

Wild Strawberry lookalike:

False Strawberry/Mock Strawberry

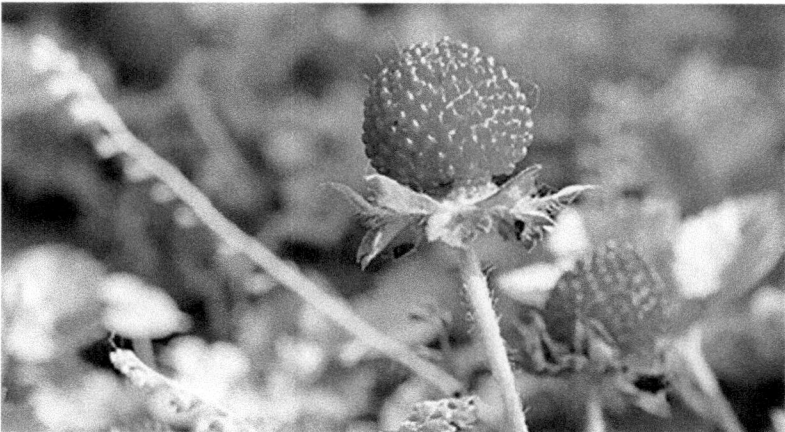

Many people are misled by the false strawberry (Potentilla indica) that holds an uncanny resemblance with wild strawberries. Still, although they may have the same sizes and even look the same, they are not toxic –just tasteless. The main difference between the lookalikes is that false strawberry has fruits pointing upwards instead of dangling from the vines, and produces yellow flowers instead of white. It also has relatively harder seeds protruding from its flesh and is a bit rounder. However, even if someone were to eat these berries accidentally, they would experience virtually no flavor and be highly disappointed. The probability that foragers might come across these is high, as these plants are invasive in the North American territory.

Chapter 7

Guide to Identifying Editable Nuts

Acorns

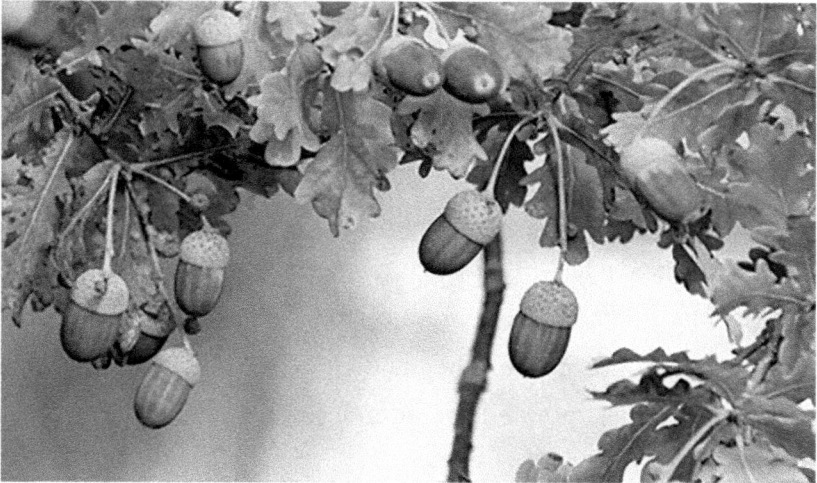

Globally, there is around 400 acorn-bearing oak species all over there world. Amongst these, 90 are native to the United States. There are two basic types of oak trees—white and red— depending on the type of oak trees they came from. All across North America, acorns can be found fallen to the ground during the fall season. After all, they can be so mass-produced that even squirrels get their fill, and leave the rest for humans to enjoy. Even though all acorns are an edible nut, they must be processed before they can be eaten. Otherwise, they taste incredibly bitter and may also damage the kidneys; this is because they are full of tannins. Foragers can remove these tannins by shelling the nuts, leeching them in a jar filled with fresh water (the water changed daily for 3 to 5 days), or grinding them into their meals. Afterward, they will be left with a mild nutty treat that can be used as a substitute for cornmeal in cornbread.

Oak trees are wildly popular and easy to identify through the presence of acorns. They look like seeds wearing a hat as they are made up of two components –the cupule (its cap) and pericarp (the hard outer shell). Although they are a very distinct nut, they have hundreds of different species, and so, the appearance of acorns varies. The colors brown, black, chestnut red and light brown are the indications of a mature acorn, while greenish-grey are not ready to be eaten yet. On the other hand, the white-colored oak is a sign of fewer tannins and a less bitter flavor, whereas red and black oaks take longer to mature and hence, produce more bitter acorns with more accumulated tannins inside. The majority of the oak trees have lobed leaves with either pointed or round knobs extending from its centerline.

American Beechnuts

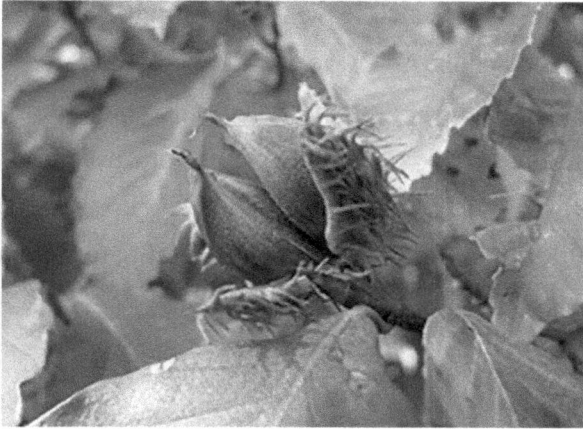

Early snow in a year increases the chances of finding beechnuts mid-winter, as they remain hidden under the blanketed snow. Typically, American beech trees produce these nutrient-dense nuts in the fall. It is okay to gobble a few beechnuts raw as they are edible, but too many of them can be toxic and cause gastric issues. Once roasted, their flavor significantly improves and becomes less toxic.

Beechnut's appearance makes them incredibly distinctive as they are brightly colored, sprawled over the forest floor. As the picture above hints, the nuts have a spiky exterior rusk. When it ripens, it pops open to reveal two small, oddly shaped nuts that have three-pointed sides. The healthiest beechnuts grow on trees with smooth grey trunks. Many times these trees have beech scale disease, invaded by pests and colonized by the fungus, after which the quality

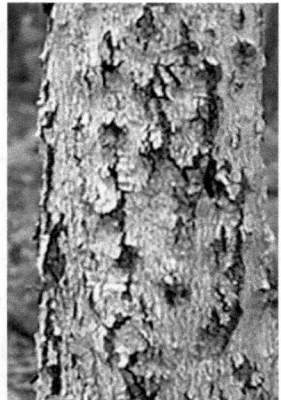

of nuts produced falls; the nuts sprouting from the tree contain empty seed shells. The disease also leaves a mark on the bark in the form of long fissures and scales. Over the trunks are 2 to 6 inches long, ovate leaves emerging from its branches. They also have points along the side and prominent veins branching out from a central vein. Dark green and glossy in summer, the leaves turn a copper-color shade in the fall. Overall, the American breech is a tall, sturdy and imposing tree, sometimes growing to 120 feet tall.

American Chestnut

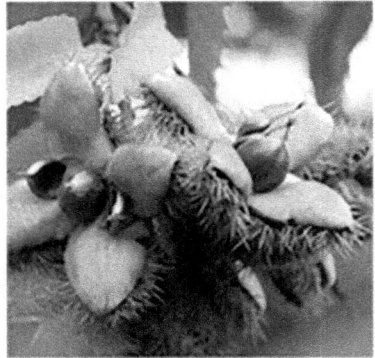

Native to North America, the American chestnut has been declared endangered for over a decade. Once, it dominated the forest species, but through a disease breakout, it has become rare. They have the strongest, resilient and decay-resistant wood amongst all North American tree species. The trees can grow up to a height of 114 feet, although that is very rare; now, it just reaches over 30 feet.

After pollination, the female flowers produce a dense, spiny husk that holds edible nuts inside. The nut has a rounded hairy tip, a sunburst base, and a pointy tip, each withholding 2 to 3 nuts about 1 inch big. They are sweet and delicious, tasting even better when roasted. The American chestnut's leaves are known to have a long, canoe shape with identifiable lance-shaped tip and forward hooked teeth. The edges are coarse, and the color is a dull, pale green.

458

American Chestnut Lookalike: Horse Chestnut

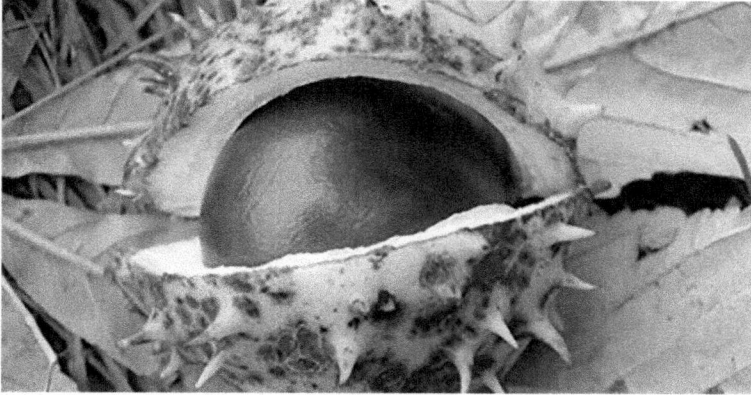

Foragers should not confuse the American chestnut with the horse chestnut as they might look really similar at first glance, especially to the untrained eye. They may seem desirable, but they are not for eating purposes, and consuming them may even cause paralysis. Not only has the nut been classified as unsafe, but even its raw bark, flowers, seeds, and leaves are toxic.

To differentiate it with its edible counterparts, its outer covering is an essential factor. Where American chestnuts are enclosed in spiny husks which have a pointed tassel on the tip, the horse chestnuts' appearance is wart-like with a bumpy, fleshy husk. Both might produce similar-looking nuts, but edible ones have a tassel (or a point), whereas the latter is smooth and round. The native horse chestnuts are sometimes also referred to as buckeyes due to their large seed resembling male deer or buck's eyes. They may develop as either a shrub or a tree, found rooted in the temperate regions of North America.

American Hezelnut

It is a native perennial shrub that stands erect up to 6 to 11 feet high. Particularly native to the Chicago region in North America, the plant forms thickets, growing best in rich, moist soils. The bark is light gray in color with a smooth texture but may become marred

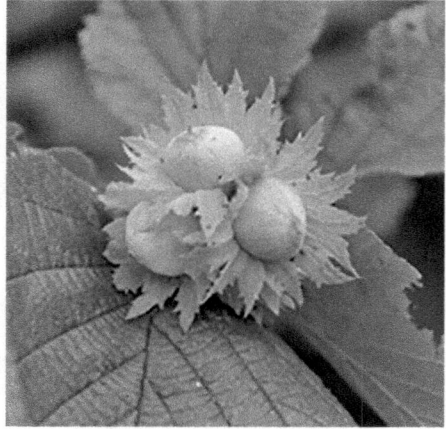

with scaly crisscross patterns as it ages. Furthermore, the light-brown twigs growing in a zigzag pattern are hairy, but young leaves are hairier. They are dark green in color with paler undersides and white hair on the veins. The leavers are either heart-shaped or rounded and turn yellow to red and purple in the fall season.

Although the male flowers (long brown catkins) may wither away after pollination, the small female flowers mature to edible nuts in September and October. These hazelnuts grow in a cluster of 2 to 5, typically enclosed in leaf-like bracts with ragged edges. Therefore, it is advisable for the foragers to wear gloves while harvesting to protect their skin from getting irritated from fine hairs. Later, foragers can eat these sweet treats raw but might want to roast t if they are looking for a sweeter, more mellow flavor.

Black Walnut

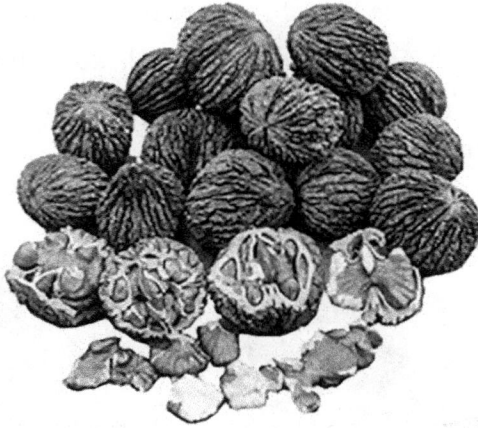

Native to North America, black walnuts can be found abundantly throughout the central-eastern United States (particularly Chicago, Illinois). It is known to favor riparian zones –the transition areas between denser woods, creeks, and rivers. Although it is edible for human beings, the black walnut tree is toxic for the plants surrounding it; it releases gases in the ground and, consequently, poisons others. Therefore, a very big giveaway of the black walnut tree, apart from it being massive (30 to 130 feet tall) and bearing rounded, hard-shelled nuts, is the yellowing or dead plants in its vicinity.

The black walnut tree, itself, is a deciduous tree, housing pinnate leaves which contain up to 25 leaflets. The leaves are toothed or serrate, consisting of an odd number of individual leaflets, all attached to a central stem. Its twigs and shoots have a chambered pith –another characteristic that confirms the tree's identity. When the nuts have matured, they drop to the ground wrapped in a spongy green husk –after the green husk degrades, it dissolves into a black color. Black walnuts taste best if they are removed from their husks as soon as possible. Many people and animals do no bother foraging for them as it takes a lot of effort for them to crack, but many consider the work worth when they taste the delicacy.

Pine Nuts

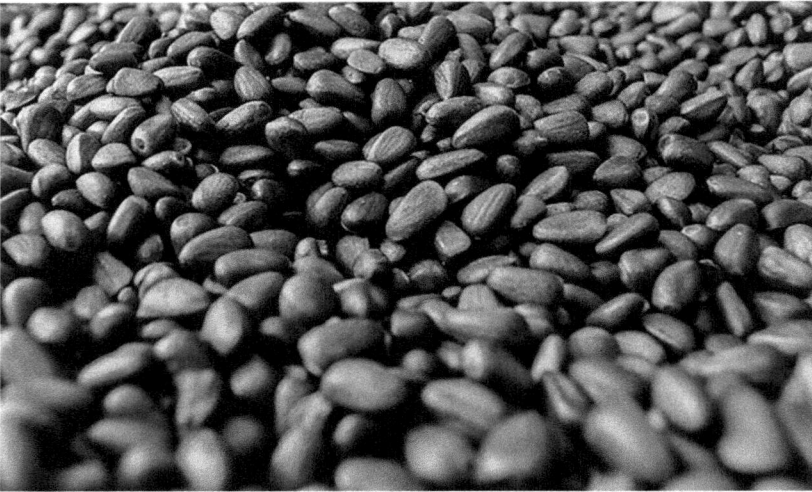

Scrubby trees bearing pine cones are spotted at high elevations in dry areas of North America. Though there are a variety of pine trees growing in the continent, only the native pinyon tree is harvested. Its nuts are large enough, unlike other pine nuts, which are not worth the effort. Pinyon pine is mostly found in the western United States, hanging off the trees in the fall and well-consumed till winters.

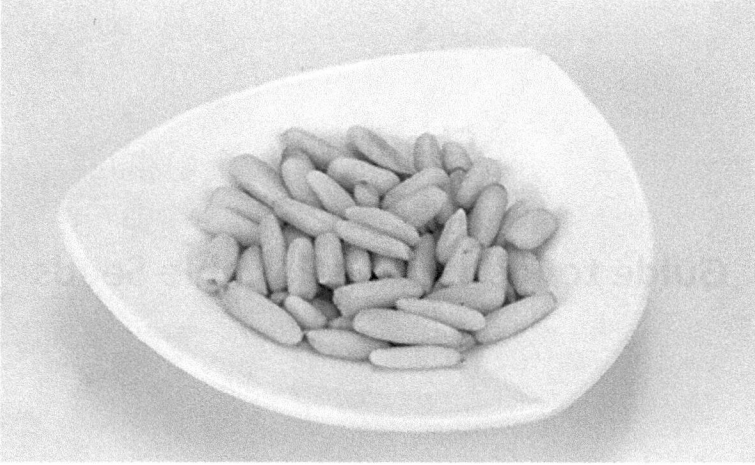

Pinyon pine is a slow-growing, evergreen tree with a rounded shape. Pinyon trees rarely grow over 20 feet and bear pine cones resembling small roses. The needles of the pinyon pine are grouped together in twos. They are flat, two-sided, and about an inch long. Within the scales of female cones are pine nuts enclosed, yielded in large amounts by the tree.

To harvest and process pine nuts is a labor-intensive process; it requires bagging the pine cones at the right time (when they are changing from green to brown); otherwise, squirrels or other rodents might beat you to it. It is important to wear gloves and old clothes at the time of harvesting; otherwise, the sap covering the cones sticks all over. Afterward, they need to be left for a few days to dry out and open up. Only then, the nuts can be carefully picked and shelled by hand. For those who love to eat these delicate and unique-flavored nuts, the tricky and laborious harvesting process is worthwhile.

Chapter 8

Guide to Identifying Editable Seeds

Alfalfa Seeds

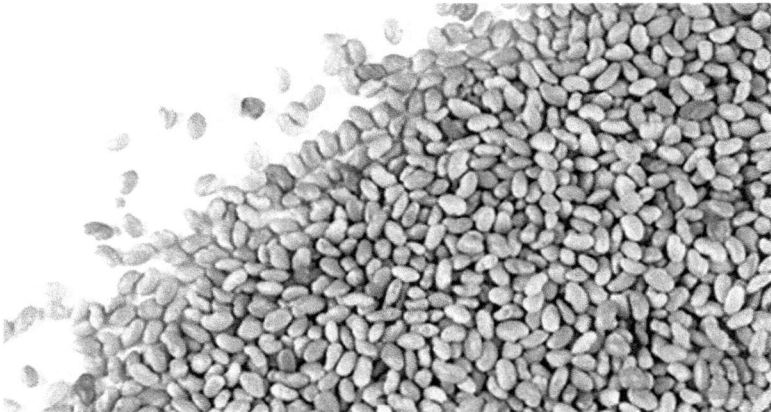

Alfalfa seeds are one of the most important legumes or forages that are used in agriculture. Their varieties are widely grown all year round and throughout the world as forage used for cattle but are found most commonly in North America. Therefore, it is considered to be the highest yielding forage plant on the continent. Alfalfa seeds can be harvested as hay, fed as a green chop, grazed in pastures, and can also be made into silage. It is a perennial legume and is well-known for its adaptability and tolerance. The plant has trifoliate leaves and flowers which range in colors from blue to violet. The seeds are kidney-shaped that are yellow, or greenish-yellow in color and turn brown as they grow older with time. To give a more precise idea, they are a shade darker than Yellow leaf clover.

Alfalfa grows best on soils that have textures ranging from fine to medium. In order to achieve the best growth results, the soil should also be medium to very well-drained. Its pH should range from neutral to high level. It can tolerate seasons of drought, but not periods of excessive flooding. It can be found growing in both wild and urban areas, including woodlands, meadows, along roadsides and abandoned areas. It prefers growing in slightly disturbed habitats and does not favor entirely untouched landscapes. Alfalfa can be planted in late spring or summer, but late summers are preferable. They must be planted approximately 0.25 to 0.5 inches, and with good contact with the soil. If it is planted in spring, it must be planted with a small grain or with grass in order to maximize tonnage in the seeding year. The seeds must be stored at low temperatures and low humidity in order to encourage their maximum growth. New plantings must not be harvested until sufficient carbohydrates are stored in the roots in order to support rapid regrowth. This is expected to happen around 60 days post-emergence. If this harvesting process is delayed for more than 60 days, the forage quality may dramatically be reduced. Alfalfa exhibits the property of autotoxicity, which means that plants older than 6 months of age, also called established plants give off compounds that prevent new alfalfa seeds from growing.

All in all, the uses of alfalfa seeds are manifold. Its leaves and young shoots are also edible. Some seeds may have an impermeable coating, which is known as hard seeds. These are impermeable to water, and these seeds may lie dormant for months or even years before germinating. They can be used later in soups as well after they have dried An appetite-stimulating tea sweetened with honey is famously made from these. On the other hand, its sprouts can be used in salads or sandwiches. These are high in protein, vitamin A, digestible energy, and minerals.

American Hornbeam Seeds

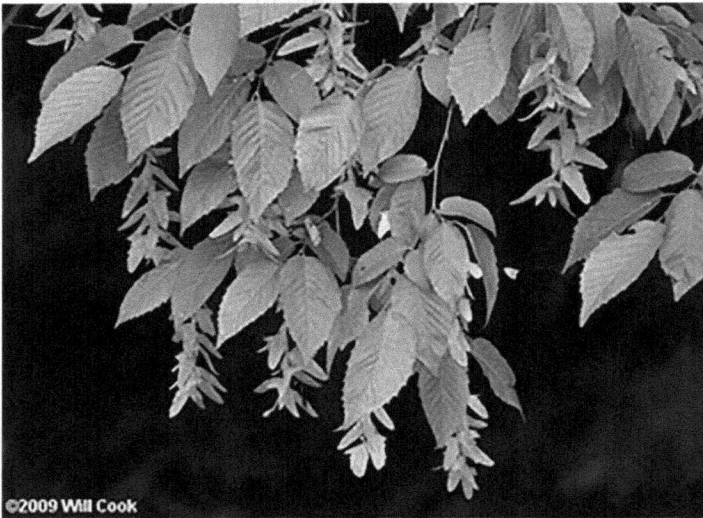
©2009 Will Cook

The American Hornbeam also goes by the names Eastern Ironwood, Eastern Hop-hornbeam, and Ostrya Virginiana. Native to North America (particularly the eastern continent), they are hardy deciduous and medium-sized, typically about 25 to 40 feet tall. They are found growing in lawns, woodland gardens, and even spotted as street trees. In the wild, the American hornbeam grows in dry soils in upland woods and rocky slopes. All over, they may have many trunks, thereby attaining the appearance of a very large shrub. Its barks are smooth, ridged, and gray, sometimes looking like as if muscles are flexed under it, therefore yielding muscle wood as another name. As it can be seen in the picture above, its leaves are oblong and tapered with depressed veins and double-teethed edges. The green flowers primarily turn to a shade of yellow in the fall, but sometimes has flashes of orange and red as well.

Most importantly, the "hops" growing on the trees have dozens of seeds encased within, as can be seen. Each tiny seed is about the size of a sunflower seed. They hang at the end of young twigs in tight clusters, enclosed in a three-lobed bract. Both the seeds and the bracts change color when they ripen –going from green to yellowish-green to light brown. Collecting seeds commences in early September, which requires a bit of an effort as the papery husk needs to be removed to extract the seeds. These seeds, depending upon the preference of foragers, be eaten raw out of hand or toasted. The trees drop these papery husks on the ground with the wind and snow, well into the winters, therefore, if one looks for them, they can be found dropped on the forest floors over the snow blanket even in midwinters. Otherwise, foragers can just shake them from branches or strip seed clusters from the twigs.

Chia Seeds

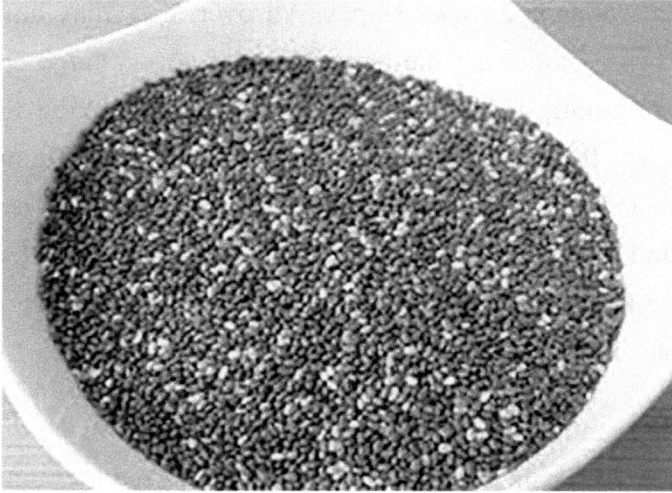

Native to North America, Chia is a flowering plant belonging to the family of mint, which is well- known and grown for the edible properties of its seeds. The Chia plant is a herbaceous plant that grows annually and can grow up to 3-feet in height. It can be easily identified from its oppositely arranged lemon-green leaves with toothed margins. Another hallmark for this plant is it's small white, blue, and purple flowers that increase the rate of self- pollination. A notable characteristic of this plant is that it is a desert plant and requires little irrigation for growth. It grows well in sandy loam soils, but it is resistant to frost as a downside.

Chia seeds extracted from these plants are oval in shape, and almost 1 mm in diameter. These seeds have a shiny and speckled seed coating that can up any shade from dark brown to gray-white in color. They have proven to be an excellent choice for organic production because they grow into plants that resist pests and diseases well.

Harvesting Chia organically is a simple process and carried out by many people at home. The seed is extracted from crushing the dried Chia flowers gently. These seeds are planted into the soil and watered in sunlight every day. Removal of weeds is necessary for a healthy yield of the plant. It must be grown in an open and relatively large space because it grows taller than most herbs and home-grown plants.

Chia seeds hold plentiful nutritional benefits. While they are rich in fiber, proteins, antioxidants, and Omega- 3 fatty acids, they can be consumed in several forms and ways. Chia pudding, smoothies, and juices, or even chia seeds mixed with yogurt, oatmeal, and as toppings on salads are common and delicious foods.

Docks

Docks are perennial plants that grow from taproots. The special feature of these plants is that their tap-like structures mean that they are resistant to drought; however, they grow the happiest in the availability of a lot of moisture. The plants grow up to be 1 to 3 feet tall in spring or late summers. Commonly found in North America, they are most spotted in neglected, disturbed ground like open fields and along roadsides.

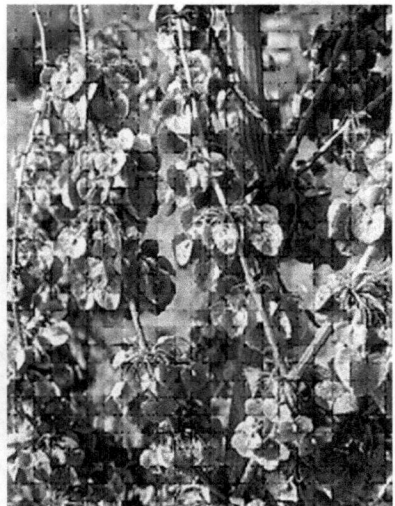

A key feature of identity for these plants is their thin sheath that covers the nodes from which the plants emerge. This is called the ocrea, and it turns brown as the plant ages or grows older. They have tall flower stalks that bear conspicuous amounts of edible seeds. The key feature to identify young plants is that their leaves are covered with mucilage. The most tender the best lemon-flavored leaves come from the young plants in which the flowers have not yet developed.

All over, dock seeds are easy to harvest, but they have a relatively short harvest season and should be gathered when they are at their peak of maturity. However, they can be reserved for later use; therefore, many people blanch or freeze them. The seeds have a slightly tart-nutty flavor after they have been roasted, which is particularly similar to rye. They can also be used in granola and crackers or can be grounded into gluten-free flour and used for baking several edibles.

Goosefoot Seeds

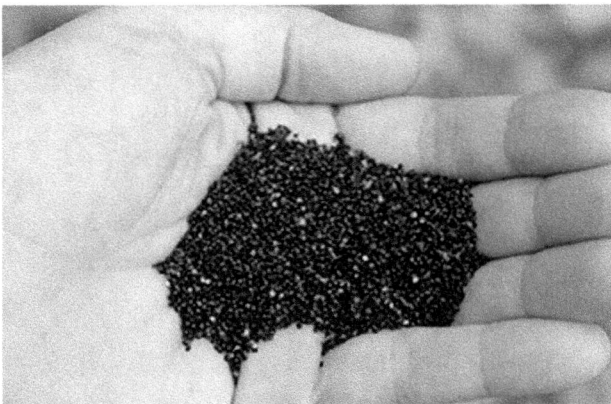

A relative of Wild Quinoa, goosefoot, is a wildly popular plant with its leaves used by American foragers in spring salads. They grow all over the United States and much of Canada as well. In fact, it is so common that all 50 states have varying species and several varieties considered native to the continent. Its name is derived from the goose-foot shaped leaves, which tastes like more flavorful and powerful spinach. Therefore, it's leaves are a notable characteristic when looking for the plant. When the heat of midsummer hits, the goosefoot plants grow taller (up to 5 feet) with tiny white seed heads sprouting from the top. The indication of the plant being mature is when it changes into a beautiful magenta hue in the fall season –that's right, the goosefoot grain is ready to be harvested.

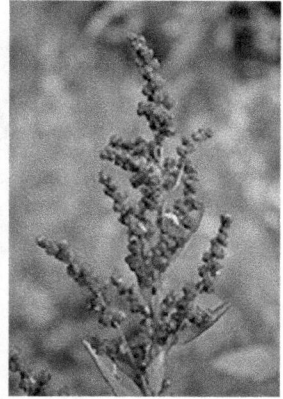

To harvest, you should place the seed clusters in the palm of your hands and gently try to strip the seed from its stalk. When you open your palms again, you will find a mixture of goosefoot grains decorating your hand. The red and green dots are the chaff, whereas the black dots are seeds that need to be separated. It could be tricky and difficult to do so, as it is not recommended to ground it into flour chaff, unlike how the dock seeds are processed. Later on, after they are separated, they can be added to pancakes, biscuits and bread batter, and soups.

471

Maple Seeds

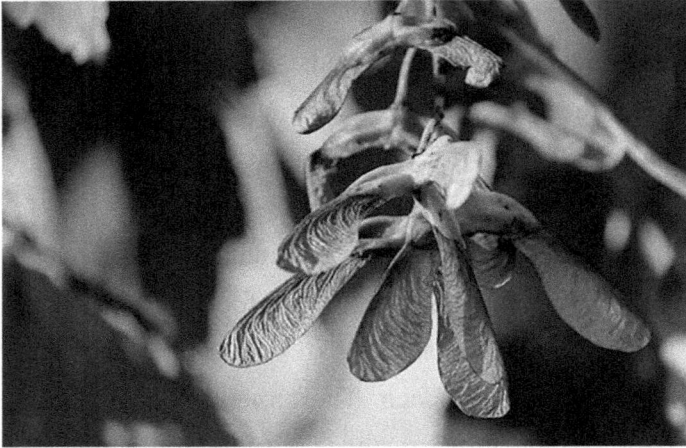

The helicopter shaped pods of maple trees are a common sight in North America. What most people do not know about these helicopter-like pods is that they enclose maple seeds which are extremely beneficial and nutritious in nature. They grow on maple trees, that are as tall as 50 meters in height. Recognized by their singular, pointed, and indented leaves. These trees produce whirling called samaras that come in pairs with their pods fused together. Inside these pods are enclosed small that are found as nutlets. In order to harvest maple, the seeds are extracted through a peeling process, as with peas. They are dried and cleaned before being sown into the soil. These are planted in spring and in a bed of 1 inch within the soil, and the seeds must be 12 inches apart. A special tip during the growing and germination phase of the seeds is to cover them with hay in order to seal in moisture. The strange quality of these seeds is that they are most delicious in spring when they are ripe and green. As they age, and in fall or winters, they become bitter. When fresh, they can be eaten in salads or as delicacies, but when bitter, they can be roasted or eaten in salads.

Ramon Seeds

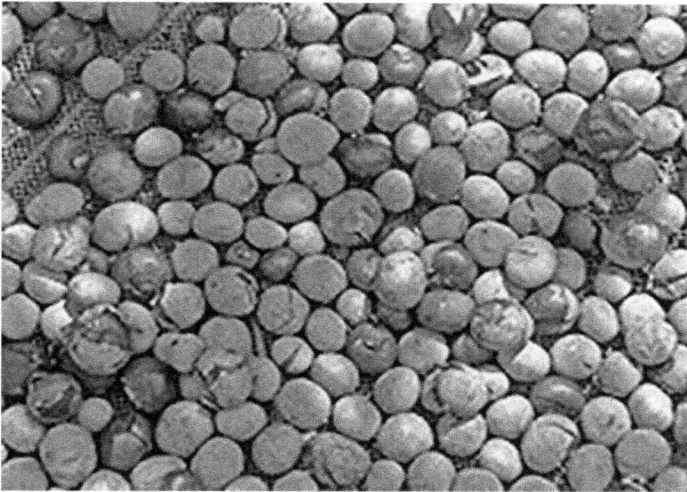

Ramón Seeds are commonly found in most parts of North America but are famously called Maya Nuts or Maya seeds in different areas. These seeds come from the fruits of the Ramon tree, which is a member of the fig family. At 130 feet tall, these trees are part of dense forest canopies. These plants are grown in vast open lands and fine-textured soils, with enough space for them to grow tall.

Its seeds are slightly larger than a coffee bean. You would notice that they are green in color when they are still present within the tree; however, they become dark brown when they are ripe. The seeds are extracted from the fruits that the tree sheds when completely ripe. Harvesting and growing these plants is an easy process, and it is used in most villages and rural areas for economic benefits and as a source of income, especially for women.

Excitingly, these seeds edible for both humans and animals. Ramon seeds are consumed by humans in several forms. They are dried and roasted into a fine powder that resembles flour and is used for baking bread and biscuits. Its powder is also similarly used as coffee, except that it does not contain any caffeine as a content. Maya nuts can be eaten fresh. However, they are most well- known for their change in flavor. When these seeds are stewed, they taste like mashed potatoes, and when they are roasted, you can easily mistake them for coffee or chocolate. The benefits of this seed are numerous. They are extremely high in doses of zinc, calcium, iron, protein, and Vitamins A, B, C, and E.

Seminole Pumpkin Seeds

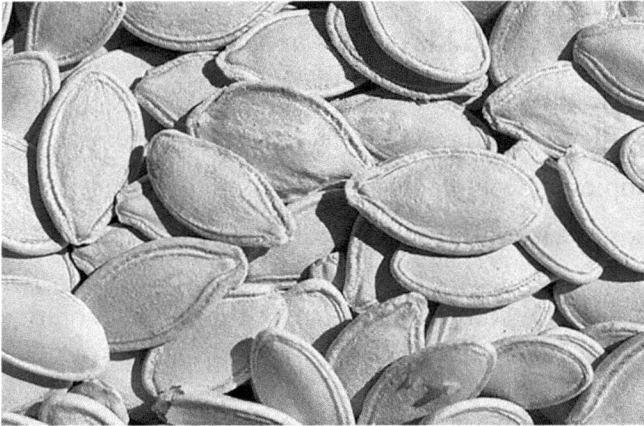

Seminole Pumpkin Seeds are found in the fruits of the Seminole Pumpkin Vines that can be found growing wild in many areas of North America. The best time for the growth of these seeds into fruits in winters and falls. They grow best in hammocks, everglades, and in abandoned cramps.

Seminole Pumpkins are similar in appearance to the famous Halloween Pumpkins, but there are some key characteristics that can be made use of in order to identify them. The vines are toothed and hairy in nature, with funnel-shaped flowers. The fruits are pear-shaped, short-necked, and orange when ripe. The seeds are enclosed in the pulpy inner flesh, and they are flat, elliptical, and white seeds, typically three-quarters of an inch in size. These are, in fact, one of the best options of planting and harvesting seeds, especially if you are a procrastinator; this is because these seeds and vines are resistant to harsh droughts as well as frosty seasons. Moreover, they also develop natural resistance to pests and diseases. They can survive while sitting on the kitchen counter for over a year, even in extreme heat and humidity.

The Seminole pumpkin seeds are extracted by cutting the fruit, usually with an ax or by softening in water. Then, they are dried and planted about 3 to 4 inches deep into the soil or at the base of growing trees. The fruits are harvested when they are completely ripe and orange. Seminole Pumpkins are famously eaten like squash. The seeds can be eaten fresh, used in soups, ground into powder, or eaten while roasted.

Tehuacan Amaranth

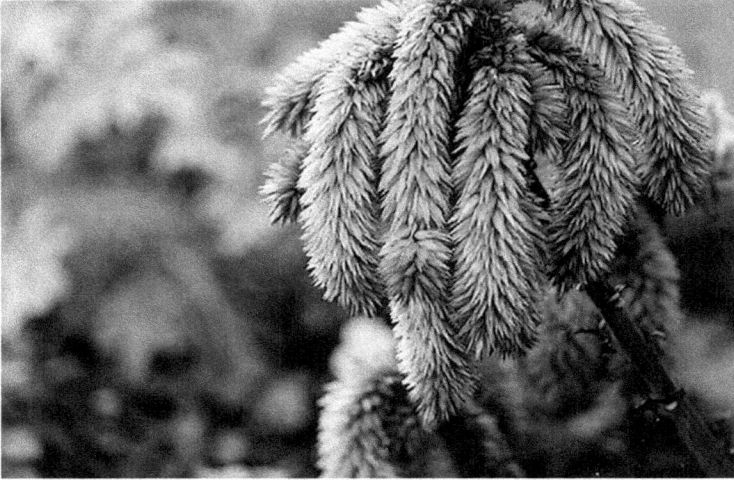

Amaranth, the anciently famous plant, has been well known for centuries and in different parts of the world for its several species and forms. In North America, the species, Tehuacan Amaranth, is of a lot of importance. This plant belongs to the Spinach family and is categorized as a flowering plant with edible seeds, commonly found growing in gardens, disturbed land, construction sites, and even roadsides. The plants are up to 2 or 3 meters in height and have large green leaves. The characteristic feature of this species that differentiates it from its other species is the magnificent flowers, which are brightly colored plumes of deep red, with pink or green nuances.

The seeds are extracted from these flowers by blowing on them when in a tilted ramp-like position so that they topple down and collect them. They are harvested only when the plants are mature and fully grown. These seeds are circular, or embryo shaped in appearance, with a shiny and beige outlook and resemble the common grain. They quickly in the rainy season and mature within a month of germination. The seeds have a small head and can be used as alternates for grains.

An interesting fact about planting Amaranth is that the plant is a self-seeder and will readily return for growth if the land is particularly disturbed. Both the seeds and leaves are of immense nutritional value, and good sources of dietary fiber, calcium, iron, and the seeds are particularly high in protein. They are nutty-tasting and can be popped, ground into flour and used to make bread or baked goods, cooked into porridge, and added into salads.

Timothy Seeds

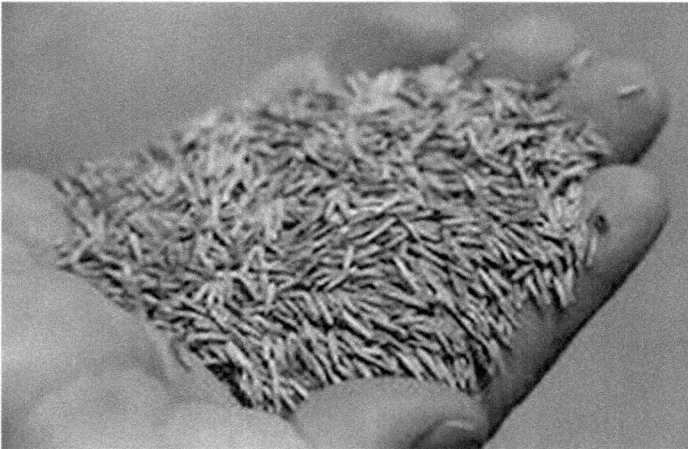

Timothy grass seeds are on top of the list of forage seeds that are common and famous in North America. These seeds are well- known for their production of flexible Timothy grass series that have numerous advantages, both agricultural and environmental. The grass is planted with legumes as nutritious forage for animals. Its plant is a flowering plant and is a light, faded green-gray color. Furthermore, they have long and hairless leaves with a characteristic twirl. These can grow up to 150 cm in height. A bulb-like base of the stem is the characteristic identification of these plants, when in the growing phase.

Seeds obtained from these plants are particularly small with an oval or elliptical shape, enclosed within glumes. They are approximately 1mm in length with a smooth texture and are white or light brown in color. The seeds are adapted to growth in a cool and humid climate. It grows best in rich soils, which have a fine texture, for example, clay looms. It also has a high tolerance from frost and ice sheets. It can be sown from spring to autumn; however, not very deep into the soil. Fertilizers, especially nitrogen, must be used frequently and in ample quantities during the growth phase. Cutting the plant as soon as the seed ripens provides nutritious forage as hay. These seeds are nutritious and edible for animals such as cattle and horses. The benefits of Timothy grass are increased nitrogen, percolation, drainage, and added nutrients.

Conclusion

We can all agree that in all of human history, three major dietary transitions occurred. Those are a transition from solely relying on hunting for meat and eating it raw, to the discovery of fire and foraging, and finally moving on to agriculture and mass food production. Humans still engage in many tasks that involve gathering multiple targets from their environment, be it take out from their favorite restaurant or their dry cleaning. So, why should picking berries or mushrooms from the environment be strange? Well, there's only one reason anyone can come up with and that because you didn't pay for it. So, there's the major argument right there. We have been offered convenience in exchange for money for way too long, and slowly, we're basically losing our basic ability to connect with nature. If we paid attention to it, foraging could become systemized as well to not just help with resource management but even deal with wastage. Food items that have a little shelf life usually go to waste even though they are good enough to eat. What is there was no demand for such products in a small town? What if a local store didn't keep herbs because people could easily pick them from parks or gardens without having to pay for them? This is the kind of society that we should be looking forward to. Not one in which there are millions of tons of food available, yet people go hungry at night just because they cannot pay for food. Our ancestors relied heavily on foraging for thousands of years before agriculture came about, and from what we have read, they got by much better.

Everyone should pick up foraging and go outdoors. There's just so much to learn and explore when you live off the land. Ask any farmer, and they'd tell you growing food is one of the best achievements of man. While foraging doesn't exactly involve growing food, it still connects you more with your environment as compared to going to a supermarket. However, foraging isn't for everyone as you have to invest a lot of time, effort, and training to harvest wild plants safely. Foraging adds adventure to your next mean, which is something you cannot expect from a trip to the supermarket. Foraging is not everyone's cup of tea. It requires time, training, and effort to learn everything that is important to know about harvesting wild fruits, vegetables, seeds, and nuts safely. In many cases, you might need to consult a local expert who can properly guide you and teach you. You might also need to gain permission to legal places meant specifically for foraging– whether it be your own land, some other private land with the owner's permission, or in public spaces. Many people think foraging is just not worth their effort and time, especially since buying fruits and vegetables at the grocery store is so much more convenient. Furthermore, navigating the ins and outs of foraging can be challenging, especially for beginners. Not only must you know what to harvest but also know if you can harvest it. For those living in cities, this can be difficult and even land you in trouble as well, so we recommend that you always follow the rules.

Foragers have been around since humans stepped foot on Earth, and even today, there are thousands and growing. Even with industrial farming has been dominating the food scene in the last century, there are those who have remained socially conscious. This is especially if you were lucky enough to group in a rural area or near farmlands. Foraging provides several things apart from getting to explore nature outside of the boxes we trap ourselves in every day. For athletes looking to remain fit by spending time outdoors, foraging presents an ample opportunity to learn about healthy food and kill two birds with one stone. If anything, foraged plants have a better nutrient profile than our regular garden varieties due to being raised in the wild. This can benefit you, your friends, and your children as well. If foraging becomes a normal practice worldwide, the next generation of kids and adults can benefit for a lifetime with the knowledge and skillsets to cope better with the upcoming economic and environmental issues. Even those with financial problems could at least have a warm meal after the end of the day. So, here's a shout out to all outdoor enthusiasts. The next time you find yourself on a camping trip, or a walk in the park with your peers, be on the lookout for different items that you could add to your dinner plate. There are incredible flavors out there just waiting to be found.

References

https://www.simonandschuster.com/books/The-Everything-Guide-to-Foraging/Vickie-Shufer/Everything/9781440525117

https://www.moneycrashers.com/foraging-guide-edible-wild-plants-food/

https://growinghealthykids.co.uk/teach-your-kids-to-forage/#:~:text=Kids%20feel%20more%20in%20control,leaves%20and%20plants%20around%20them.

https://www.fourseasonforaging.com/blog/2019/3/19/foraging-legality

https://www.rootwell.com/blogs/foraging-beginners

https://www.thewondersmith.com/blog/2019/introtoforaging

https://scanmarker.com/2019/09/25/the-top-10-most-useful-gadgets-for-professionals/

https://www.hongkiat.com/blog/high-tech-camping-gadgets/

https://www.doyou.com/4-reasons-why-everyone-should-know-how-to-cook/

https://www.countryliving.com/uk/wildlife/countryside/a3009/foraging-beginner-tips/

https://www.countryliving.com/uk/wildlife/countryside/a3009/foraging-beginner-tips/

https://en.wikipedia.org/wiki/Scoutcraft#:~:text=Scoutcraft%20is%20a%20term%20used,country%20and%20sustain%20themselves%20independently.

https://www.healthline.com/health/most-powerful-medicinal-plants#We-scoured-through-histories-of-herbal-studies-for-you

https://blog.mybalancemeals.com/health/health-tips/8-natural-aspirin-alternatives/

https://webecoist.momtastic.com/2008/09/30/most-powerful-potent-medicinal-medical-plants-in-nature/

https://www.redbubble.com/shop/foraging+accessories

https://gallowaywildfoods.com/foraging-equipment-fungi-knives/

https://www.modern-forager.com/products/modern-forager-mushroom-hunting-knife/

https://www.sciencedirect.com/topics/agricultural-and-biological-sciences/manual-harvesting

http://www.bbc.com/travel/story/20120510-the-art-of-urban-foraging

http://www.takepart.com/article/2014/07/09/public-fruit-trees/

https://foodtank.com/news/2018/12/opinion-five-zero-food-waste-bloggers-you-should-know-about/

http://paulkirtley.co.uk/2013/survival-foraging-a-realistic-approach/

http://www.takepart.com/article/2014/07/09/public-fruit-trees/

https://ir.lawnet.fordham.edu/cgi/viewcontent.cgi?article=2740&context=ulj

https://www.khanacademy.org/humanities/big-history-project/early-humans/how-did-first-humans-live/v/bhp-from-foraging-to-food-shopping

https://www.cranberries.org/

https://www.encyclopedia.com/plants-and-animals/plants/plants/horse-chestnut

https://www.moneycrashers.com/foraging-guide-edible-wild-plants-food/

http://www.eattheweeds.com/

https://leafyplace.com/types-of-berries/

https://www.healthline.com/nutrition/wild-berries#1

https://practicalselfreliance.com/winter-foraging/

https://foodtank.com/news/2016/07/indigenous-foods-historically-and-culturally-important-to-north-americ/

https://practicalselfreliance.com/edible-wild-berries-fruits/

http://www.eattheweeds.com/cucurbita-muschata-seminole-edible-2/

https://www.fourseasonforaging.com/blog/2018/2/19/crabapples-the-winter-sweet-tart

www.ingramcontent.com/pod-product-compliance
Lightning Source LLC
Chambersburg PA
CBHW062110020426
42335CB00013B/908